Cosmetic Surgery

Cosmetic Surgery

The Cutting Edge of Commercial Medicine in America

DEBORAH A. SULLIVAN

RUTGERS UNIVERSITY PRESS
New Brunswick, New Jersey, and London

Second paperback printing, 2004

Library of Congress Cataloging-in-Publication Data

Sullivan, Deborah A., 1947–
    Cosmetic surgery : the cutting edge of commercial medicine in America /
Deborah A. Sullivan.
      p. cm.
    Includes bibliographical references and index.
    ISBN 0-8135-2859-3 (cloth: alk. paper) — ISBN 0-8135-2860-7 (pbk. : alk. paper)
    1. Surgery, Plastic. 2. Surgery, Plastic—Economic aspects. 3. Surgery,
Plastic—Marketing. 4. Surgery, Plastic—Social aspects. I. Title.

RD119.S85 2000
617.9'5—dc21

                                       00-039028

British Cataloging-in-Publication data for this book is available from the British Library

Manufactured in the United States of America

Contents

Acknowledgments

This book forced me to think about commercialism, not only in medicine, but also in everyday life. The imperative of commercialism has provided me a material standard of living that is the envy of much of the world's population, but the most important aspects of my quality of life have not been met by commercial goods and services. The national movement to commercialize education with public money makes me realize how blessed I was to be educated by the Sisters of St. Joseph. Faced with classes of fifty or more students and no assistants, they persistently pushed us to acquire the fundamental skills needed for adulthood. They never received a penny for their efforts. Their motivation was much stronger than commercial. I hope they are justly rewarded.

I also must acknowledge a man who, over the course of many raucous Sunday afternoon debates with me and my siblings, taught me that you need facts, not opinions, to make a convincing argument and that no issue is as simple as it seems on the surface. He motivated me to learn more about social issues, forced me to do my Latin without a trot, tutored me in math, corrected my misspellings, and criticized every paper I wrote. Every child should be so fortunate.

This book could not have been written without another non-commercial service—libraries. I have been helped by many librarians in the course of this research. One, Madeleine Mullin, deserves special mention. She oversees the American Society of Plastic and

Reconstructive Surgeons' Archives at Harvard's Countway Library and was immensely helpful to me. Countway's comprehensive collection of medical journals was also invaluable.

Several graduate students helped with literature searches, including Kitty Coons and John Parker. Tanya Neiri also helped with a survey of physicians involved in cosmetic surgery. These data will be published elsewhere. These and many other graduate and undergraduate students, family members, friends, and a few members of the Society for Women in Sociology helped by sending me cosmetic surgery ads from around the country.

The input of a few colleagues deserves separate mention. Rose Weitz read early drafts of some chapters and helped me clarify my focus. Mary Laner read the full manuscript with her sharp editorial eye and unflagging encouragement. An anonymous reviewer offered some excellent suggestions.

I would like to thank my family for support. They have been tolerant of my occasional AWOL status when I lost track of the time. They have had to endure the embarrassment of having friends discover their mother reads books with titles like *Mutilating the Body: Identity in Blood and Ink* and *Tattoos and Bad Boys.* They did not complain too much when stacks of cosmetic surgery ads covered an imaginary map of the United States on the family room floor for about a month. A special thanks goes to my husband, who, despite his claims that he knew nothing about this subject, came up with the best metaphor in the book.

Introduction

The pursuit of beauty is big business in modern societies. Americans spend $20 billion annually on products advertised to enhance appearance. Yet, for many, this is not enough. Dissatisfaction with personal appearance is widespread, particularly among women. Surveys indicate that one-half are unhappy with one or more aspects of their bodies (Cash 1997). They would like to change, rather than merely enhance, their appearance. More than one-third would like to alter their thighs. One fourth would like to change their buttocks, and about the same proportion would like to erase their facial wrinkles. Nearly one in five want different breasts and one in seven want different noses. Although American men do not express as much discontent as women with their personal appearance, about one-fourth would like to modify one or more of their own body parts.

The preceding statistics come from a national survey, sponsored not by a cosmetics firm, a weight-loss company, nor a health-club chain, but by a physicians' professional organization—the American Society of Plastic and Reconstructive Surgeons (1998a). Beauty has become a medical business as an increasing number of men and women turn to doctors to change their appearance. Estimates of cosmetic medical procedures in the United States range from 4.6 million (American Society for Aesthetic Plastic Surgery 2000) to 4.9 million per year (American Academy of Cosmetic Surgery 2000). If skin treatments involving Botox, peels, and injections of collagen, fat, and fibril are excluded, the annual number of remaining cosmetic surgery procedures in recent years is still over 2 million. Cosmetic surgery has become a modern body custom.

In the chapters that follow I examine some changes in the American cultural context that have made cosmetic surgery a modern body custom and a commercial medical practice. Although patients are disproportionately female and cosmetic surgery is often used to intensify the "gendered" appearance of bodies, it is not an exclusively feminine custom, nor an exclusively gender custom. Nevertheless, cosmetic surgery inscribes our gendered beliefs about appearance, physical fitness, and age in our flesh. It personifies the social, psychological, and economic value we place on an attractive appearance, regardless of gender. It embodies advances in medical technology and the professional authority and autonomy that physicians achieved in the early part of the twentieth century. It incarnates the image-obsessed consumerism and competitive free-market economy of the late twentieth century. In the process of constructing modern social bodies, cosmetic surgery not only puts the physical well-being of patients at risk, it also puts the unified organization and service ethic of physicians at risk, jeopardizing the foundation of their professional authority and autonomy.

This book is neither a consumer guide to cosmetic surgery nor an ethnographic account of the body custom. Rather, it presents an attempt to understand what factors contributed to the emergence and growth of demand for this medical practice, the supply of practitioners offering it, and the implications of its subsequent commercialism for medicine. In retrospect, this project started in the early 1990s when I noticed several articles about cosmetic surgery in my daughters' teenage magazines. The journalists seemed to be enthusiastically endorsing surgical solutions for generic teenage anxiety about appearance. My concern about this message opened my eyes to the extensive number of advertisements for cosmetic surgery in my local area and the "infomercial" quality of its coverage in the news media and magazines. The mail brought invitations to community seminars on the subject held in rented hotel function rooms and at prestigious medical centers. I attended some. It was difficult for me to reconcile watching physicians promote elective surgery to embellish a normal appearance with the history of medicine's struggle for a unified organization, cultural legitimacy, professional authority, and autonomy, a struggle that I was teaching in my sociology of health and illness classes. Cosmetic surgery seemed to be a throwback to the commercialism of the turn-of-the-century medical free market that the American Medical Association had succeeded in eradicating in its campaign to professionalize medicine and upgrade the quality of health care.

How had cosmetic surgery become a modern body custom? For the most part, my research was conducted in the reverse order of its presentation in this book. I began by trying to discern the cultural ideology about cosmetic surgery with a systematic analysis of the cosmetic surgery content in women's magazines in the 1980s. Later I extended the analysis to 1995 to capture the impact of the breast implant crisis on the media for chapter 7. I collected the advertisements used in chapter 6 at the beginning and end of the 1990s. These two chapters examine the overt and implied media messages about cosmetic surgery and consider the consequences of its commercialism for medical judgement and practitioners' potential conflict of interest.

A few of the magazine articles alluded to an intraprofessional conflict over cosmetic surgery. To learn more about this conflict, I examined nearly three decades of editorials, letters to the editor, and relevant articles in specialty medical journals for plastic surgeons, otolaryngologists, dermatologists, ophthalmologists, and maxillofacial surgeons. I read all issues of the plastic surgeons' newsletter through the summer of 1997, available at the American Society of Plastic and Reconstructive Surgeons' archives at Harvard's Countway Library. I read histories commissioned by this organization, the American Academy of Facial Plastic and Reconstructive Surgery, the American Academy of Ophthalmology, and the American Academy of Otolaryngology—Head and Neck Surgery. I also read the three-volume transcript of the 1989 congressional hearings on cosmetic surgery and the 1990 hearings on silicone breast implants, as well as the Federal Trade Commission documents related to its antitrust complaint against the American Society of Plastic and Reconstructive Surgeons. Finally, I examined statistical data on physicians collected by the American Medical Association and the U.S. Census Bureau. The information from these sources forms the basis for the discussion of the economic and political changes that have facilitated the growth and commercialization of cosmetic surgery, discussed in chapter 4; created the intraprofessional conflict, discussed in chapter 5; and led to the reappearance of physician advertising, discussed in chapter 6. I also discovered that actions taken by physicians and their professional organizations, in response to economic and political changes and the resulting intraprofessional conflict, have shaped the ideology about cosmetic surgery presented in the advertisements and women's magazines in ways designed to promote patient demand.

Chapter 3 provides a historical overview of the technological innovations in medicine that made cosmetic surgery possible. As in other occupations, there is a close connection between technological innovation and evolving specialization in medicine's division of labor. Technological innovations in reconstructive surgery created the opportunity for broadening the definition of what constitutes a medical problem to include appearance. In the context of social change in beliefs, values, relationships, sex roles, and economic and social institutions, this opportunity had the force of an imperial fiat. The historical background provides a context for understanding the deep roots of the problems that cosmetic surgery presents for the medical profession. It illuminates cosmetic surgery's inherent commercialism and its often difficult relationship with noncommercial medicine. It reveals the long-standing importance of women's magazines for conveying changing medical ideology about cosmetic surgery and promoting demand. Finally, it explains the origin of the current official medical ideology that cosmetic surgery can be justified as a mental health treatment.

There is no comprehensive medical history of cosmetic surgery available at the time of this writing, although two recently published books offer partial histories and alternative theories about the growth of demand for this modern custom. Elizabeth Haiken's *Venus Envy: A History of Cosmetic Surgery* (1997) offers a fascinating account of early twentieth-century American "beauty surgeons" and their struggle for respectability. Her primary focus is on facial surgery in the context of popular culture. She attributes the growth in cosmetic surgery to patients' relentless demands for medical help with appearance for reasons that range from aging to racial and ethnic stigmas. She also traces the history of physicians' eventual willingness to accept cosmetic surgery as a legitimate treatment for an inferiority complex.

Sander Gilman's *Making the Body Beautiful: A Cultural History of Aesthetic Surgery* (1999) also draws on literature, art, and film, as well as historical medical articles. Like Haiken, he attributes the growth of cosmetic surgery to patient demand originating in a desire to be happy. Unlike Haiken, he argues that patients are primarily driven by a desire to pass themselves off as members of the dominant social group. His more narrow interpretation of motivation may stem from

his more narrow focus on rhinoplasty among Jews and other stigmatized groups in the first seven chapters, although he devotes his last
two chapters to transsexual surgery and "rejuvenation" procedures.

Rather than focusing on the influences of popular culture, which
has been done well by these historians, I review, in chapter 2, the social science research on the consequences of appearance for both men
and women in order to discuss the causes of patient demand for cosmetic surgery. The findings suggest that people who seek cosmetic surgery are responding rationally to measurable social, psychological, and
economic rewards and penalties based on the dominant ideals and
beliefs about appearance, discussed in chapter 1 along with the concept of "social bodies." Chapter 2 also considers the impact of changes
in occupational structure, employment stability, women's labor-force
participation, and marital trends on the intensification of concern with
appearance.

The chapter sequence reflects my belief that patient demand for
cosmetic surgery in response to cultural pressures to be attractive is a
necessary, but insufficient, explanation for its emergence as a modern body custom. Changes within medicine also must be considered.
Cosmetic surgery could not exist without the participation of physicians. Medical licensure gives physicians not only monopoly over the
practice of medicine, but also the legal authority to define the scope
of medical practice. Not many physicians were willing to do cosmetic
procedures in the first half of the twentieth century. After considerable internal debate, mainstream medicine subsumed cosmetic surgery
as a medical practice. This decision was not without trepidation about
the potential consequences. The commercialization that has since
emerged for cosmetic surgery affirms the legitimacy of early opponents'
concerns about including cosmetic surgery within medicine. The last
chapter considers implications of commercialized cosmetic surgery for
patients' physical well-being and for professional ethics, authority, and
autonomy. More generally, it considers whether the problems created
by commercialized cosmetic surgery might stand as a harbinger for all
commercialized medicine.

Cosmetic Surgery

1 | Social Bodies
Tightening the Bonds of Beauty

Cosmetic surgery is a modern variation of a practice as old as humankind. Every culture has some customs that prescribe deliberately changing a body's natural appearance (Brain 1979). The methods, however, are diverse and particular to a culture at a specific period of time. Paints, for example, are used to decorate bodies in many cultures, but the pigments, patterns, permanency, and purpose of each culture's body customs vary widely. Only a nineteenth-century Bedouin woman could appreciate the eroticism of painting the whites of a man's eyes blue. While she would have regarded her own culture's customs as highly "civilized," she probably would have thought the full body designs of Aboriginal Australians, American Indians, and Africans savage. Like eighteenth-century European explorers, she might have considered the tattooing and tooth-blackening in the Pacific region bizarre, and found the deeply carved black spirals and curves on Maori faces frightening and repulsive. It is no more likely that she could have discerned the beauty intended by the African and South American tribes who create elaborate patterns of raised scars, insert large lip plates and ear and nose plugs, and file teeth to sharp points. Nor is it likely that she could have appreciated the charm of Chinese women's bound "lotus" feet, Padaung women's elongated necks, or Western women's constricted waists during the Victorian era and augmented breasts in recent decades. Instead, in the implausible circumstance that a nineteenth-century Bedouin

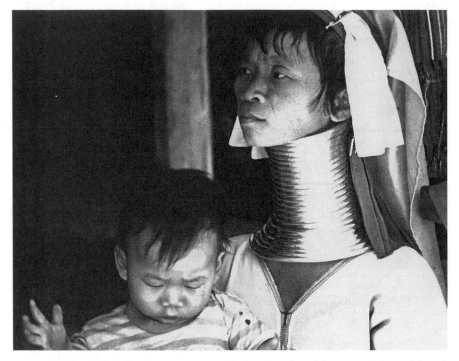

Figure 1.1. Padaung woman and baby. *Reprinted by permission of Derek Brook-Wavell.*

woman was exposed to such body customs, she probably would have regarded them as barbaric mutilations, much as contemporary Americans' view of female circumcision, which she might have considered normal.

The diversity of body customs has led anthropologists (e.g., Douglas 1970; Strathern 1996) to conclude that a body is both a physical and a symbolic artifact, forged by nature and by culture at a particular moment in history. Social institutions, ideology, values, beliefs, and technology transform a physical body into a social body. The resulting social body bears the imprint of the more powerful elements of its cultural context. Bodies, therefore, provide important clues to the mechanics of society.

This chapter provides a brief overview of the social nature of bodies and the feminine and masculine standards that have evolved in the context of rapid cultural and social change over the last two centuries and concludes with a definition of cosmetic surgery and some statistics on the incidence of this modern body custom.

Social Bodies

There are many well-documented examples of the cultural construction of a social body. Although some body customs may be merely decorative, many, if not most, have social significance. Cultures in which female circumcision is common are strongly patriarchal and pronatalist. Women in these traditional cultures are believed to be weak and incapable of controlling their sexual urges. They are allowed little contact with men outside their families and are expected to hide their bodies from public view. Their social roles are circumscribed to child care and domestic functions. They receive little education and are economically dependent on men and politically powerless. They are socialized by their mothers to believe that removal of external female genitalia is a religious obligation that promotes purity, cleanliness, and fertility and that unexcised women are unattractive and beastly. Their identities as desirable women depend on the submission of their physical bodies to the dictates of social norms. The custom embodies their inferior status.

As female circumcision illustrates, the body can be a site for the expression of power in a culture. It also is used to communicate group membership, individual status, and social identity, along with associated beliefs and values. The body is often ritually modified in connection with major life transitions. In the Australian Aboriginal culture, for example, one or two front teeth are removed at puberty. Some time later boys are painted white, secluded, and circumcised to symbolize their passage into the world of men. At the end of the ceremony, they are painted red to celebrate their reentry into society as young men with all the corresponding rights and expectations of their new status. In some tribes young men undergo a subincision ceremony in which their urethra is split open before they marry and assume full adult male rights. Rites of passage between life stages in many other cultures are marked by ritualized patterns of scarification, piercing, and tattooing. These same techniques are used to proclaim more permanent kinds of social status, such as gender and social class, as are head molding and other body modifications.

Using the body to communicate power, group membership, individual status, and social identity is not limited to exotic non-Western societies. It is ubiquitous in modern societies as well. American sailors, prisoners, bikers, and other gang members have tattooed their bodies throughout most of the twentieth century. Clinton Sanders (1989) argues that they use this particular body custom, considered vulgar

by most middle-class, middle-aged Americans, to proclaim their resistance to conventional social norms of appearance and behavior. Their
preference for death symbols, predatory animals, insulting and sala-
cious images further enhances their rebellious statement.

After the mid-1960s the shock value of tattoos made them popular
among some younger artistic individuals looking for attention and innovative, creative modes of expression. By the 1980s they were de
rigueur among heavy metal and rap performers seeking a following
among adolescents and young adults based on flaunting the conventional values and beliefs of their parents and other authority figures.
Punks, freaks, Goths, skinheads, stoners, tweakers, and other disaffected
young adults who identified with the counterculture heroes of their
generation went to shops with names like Hierarchy, Crawling Squid,
and Pigments of Imagination to record their sense of alienation on their
bodies.

The meaning of tattoos changed in the 1990s. They became a
badge of youth. Professional athletes, middle-class college students,
blue-collar workers, and even some suburban housewives marked their
bodies with tribal patterns, Kanji lettering, and sexy butterflies and
flowers. As the shock value of tattoos declined, the most alienated subgroups added other forms of body modifications to advertise their con-
tempt for middle-class conventions. They pierced their ears, noses,
eyebrows, lips, tongues, nipples, navels, and genitalia with safety pins,
barbells, studs, and various rings. These cultural pioneers established
Internet news groups to share information about techniques, complications, public reaction, and erotic effects. Pop singers and other
media celebrities adopted less extreme versions of this new body custom to advertise their hip identity. High school girls turned nose studs
and navel rings into a fashion statement, undermining their deviance
value. Those seeking a body symbol of resistance capable of generating strong public revulsion experimented with more extreme forms
of self-stigmatization, such as scalp implants and scarification, to proclaim their marginalized status.

Tattooing and piercing at the end of the twentieth century appear to have much in common with previous fashion fads that visu-
ally differentiated each young generation over the course of the
twentieth century, although some cultural observers (e.g., Polhemus
and Randall 1996) find deeper meaning in these trends. They suggest
the practices express a yearning for continuity, community, and commitment in a fragmented postmodern culture where ritual is rare and

anomie prevails. Tattooing and piercing offer more permanent ways of recording life transitions and one's place in society.

All body customs, whether temporary, like tweezing eyebrows and clipping nose hair, or more permanent, like tattoos and cosmetic surgery, are forms of self-creation. They are an effort to achieve a desired identity and connection with a reference group—marginal, hip, or mainstream. The process of reincarnation is universal.

Kim Hewitt (1997) additionally argues that body customs, particularly painful ones, can be used as part of a self-chosen health ritual. She theorizes that the physiological effects of pain can stimulate at least a temporary reprieve from numbing feelings of alienation (118). The acute awareness of feeling alive induced by pain has the potential to replace psychological fragmentation with holistic integration and a euphoric feeling of self-mastery. She claims that young women who starve and cut their bodies, like the punks and other marginalized subgroups who customize their bodies in extreme ways, are not only rebelling against societal constrictions, they also are trying to reclaim control of their bodies and establish individuality and autonomy. Other body customs, including female bodybuilding (Heywood 1998) and cosmetic surgery (Davis 1995), have been similarly interpreted as methods of psychological healing and cultural empowerment.

Those with a more Foucauldian perspective, such as Susan Bordo (1993, 1997), argue that such "disciplinary" body customs are outward manifestations of internalized cultural oppression. The discipline comes from an awareness of prevailing values, beliefs, norms and voluntary self-surveillance. Consequently, the sense of power experienced by disciplining one's own body, whether to resist prevailing cultural dictates with tattoos and piercings or successfully conform to them with diets and cosmetic surgery, is merely a personal achievement that lacks political effect to change the culture. Instead, as Rosemary Gillespie (1996) points out, customs such as cosmetic surgery perpetuate wider social inequalities.

This debate raises perennial philosophical questions about the nature of social control and the extent of free will. It also raises contemporary concerns that interpreting personal behavior as victimization deprives individuals of agency and castes them as gullible cultural dupes. My own perspective is similar to that of Bordo. Respect for the right of competent adults to make decisions about their own bodies should not blind us to the impact of the larger cultural and social context in which personal choices occur. My aim is to bring the structural aspects of this context, aspects that construct cosmetic surgery, into sharper focus. This larger cultural and social context influences individual body choices, gives them social meaning, and makes some, like cosmetic surgery, common enough to be considered body customs.

When powerful cultural ideologies and social institutions change, body standards and customs change. This is clearly evident in the changing standards for feminine and masculine bodies over the last two centuries.

The Changing Ideal
Femininity

Body customs change as social institutions, relationships, values, beliefs, and technology change. Lois Banner's 1983 history, *American Beauty,* reveals how changes in these social factors in the nineteenth and early twentieth centuries are linked to changes in female appearance. The homespun, republican idealism of the eighteenth century valued simplicity and naturalness in all things, including appearance. In contrast, the paragon of beauty in the rapidly industrializing nineteenth century was an ethereal, willowy, young woman dressed lavishly in layers of fabrics and trims. Her milk-white skin, small "bee-stung" mouth, and hourglass figure were achieved by using homemade cosmetics, eating chalk and arsenic, drinking vinegar, and wearing a tightly laced corset. The ideal waist was a mere eighteen inches, small enough for a man to encircle with his hands. After the middle of the century padding was added to bosoms and hips to further exaggerate the desired feminine contour. Later, bustles highlighted women's buttocks. Such heavy, constrictive clothing made work, exercise, and eating difficult. It also undermined women's health by creating musculoskeletal problems and displacing internal organs. The custom persisted, despite attempts at dress reform by feminists and physicians, because it was imbued with social meaning.

The fragile delicacy of genteel women in the nineteenth century maintained the gender and class hierarchy in a time of rapid social change. Their idleness and opulent dress were status symbols for the men who supported them. Female invalidism assumed cult status. As Thorstein Veblen noted in his 1899 *Theory of the Leisure Class*, middle-class women enhanced the upward mobility prospects of their men in the economic expansion of industrialization by imitating the ornamental function of upper-class women. At the same time, by striving for spiritual refinement rather than personal comfort, these women reinforced the Victorian belief that beauty embodied purity, piety, self-denial, domesticity, and submissiveness.

Social change, including industrialization, commercialization, secularization, immigration, the demand for female labor, and suffrage, eventually eroded the restraints of Victorian ideology and body customs. At the turn of the twentieth century, the stronger, more athletic ideal of the patrician Gibson girl, who still wore a corset, democratized into the unbound, energetic, urban flapper of the 1920s. Her idealized, youthful, boyish shape, bobbed hair, loose, light-weight dress, and uncovered limbs embodied women's new freedoms. The emerging commercial beauty industries nurtured the new consumer ideology that every woman could be beautiful, if she purchased the right cosmetic products, hairstyle, and clothes.

The Great Depression ended the youthful exuberance of the Roaring Twenties, but not the growth of the commercial beauty industries. Necessity and opportunity continued to pull women into the paid labor force until the end of World War II. Broad shoulders came into vogue, underscoring women's assumption of "masculine" roles and competencies. When the servicemen came home, however, the still dominant traditional gender and class ideologies dictated that middle-class wives and mothers relinquish their wartime jobs. A return to a softer, more curvaceous standard of beauty for the average woman followed. Girdles, brassieres, and falsies were used to mold the modern body. Unlike her nineteenth-century predecessors, a fifties beauty in her form-fitting skirts and sweaters and pool-side tan exuded robust health and restrained sexuality, amplified by the liberal use of commercial cosmetic and hair products. By this time the latter included bleaches, dyes, and permanent waves that changed the hair itself, not just the style.

Feminine body norms continued to change. The Civil Rights movement encouraged an affirmation of racial and ethnic differences in appearances. The Vietnam War protest was literally painted on young bodies. These same bodies were refashioned by rebellion against other forms of perceived cultural hypocrisy and injustice, ranging from repressive sexual mores and gender roles to the industrial and municipal defiling of nature. Young women in the late 1960s and 1970s shunned their mothers' restrictive undergarments, stylized coiffures, conspicuous makeup, and matronly bodies. The more radical feminists and eco-activists also shunned their custom of removing hair from legs and underarms and wearing makeup. A younger, thinner, more "natural," sexually available appearance became the norm. To look good required more disciplinary effort. Dieting, jogging, tennis, and aerobics became popular activities. Demand for cosmetic surgery grew. When these young women began to flood into the labor force, pantsuits adapted from menswear overtook miniskirts and granny dresses. After affirmative action policies produced a significant number of women with professional degrees and nontraditional career aspirations in the business-oriented 1980s, pantsuits evolved into broad-shouldered "power dressing," ideally worn over sexy undergarments and firm, fit bodies that spent time cross training and working out at the local gym.

How closely a woman's physical body approximated the beauty standard of a period was more readily apparent in the twentieth century than in the nineteenth century. Modern clothing was far more revealing of the underlying body than Victorian clothing, and secularization undermined the value placed on purity and piety as components of female beauty. As a result, the physical body, rather than the more holistically conceived, clothed person of the nineteenth century, became the basis for judgements about appearance. This transition is reflected in the history of beauty pageants.

Unlike the young women who hoped to be selected queen of the May and similar festivals in previous times, contestants in the first Miss America competition in 1921 were required to don bathing suits and strut in front of judges. The controversial practice continues today. In an attempt to assuage critics, talent and interview assessments were added to create a composite score. Nevertheless, many articulate and talented beauty contestants turn to physicians to "correct" perceived flaws in their physical appearance. They believe that the modern standard of beauty, discussed in more detail in chapter 2, is too narrow to allow even minor imperfections to show and there is little room to hide them in a bathing suit. The focus on the ever more visible body has heightened the importance of physical appearance for every woman, not just professional beauties, and contributed to the rise in demand for cosmetic surgery.

Masculinity

With the exception of head and facial hair styles, male body norms have varied less than female norms over the last two centuries. Masculinity, with rare exception, has been associated with power, strength, and domination and symbolized by muscularity. Nevertheless, there has been variation in the degree of muscularity deemed ideal. Over the course of the nineteenth century, industrialization increased affluence and the proportion of men who could avoid physically taxing labor and malnutrition. Prosperity made a middle-aged "spread" and softer bodies more common, not only in the upper class, but also in the growing middle class. The more fashion conscious corseted their girth. Others adopted new methods of body discipline promoted by the physical culture movement.

The physical culture movement grew out of Lamarckian ideology in the early part of the century (Dutton 1995). This ideology led to concern that the increasingly sedentary lives of the middle and upper classes would result in cultural degeneracy and erode the physical fitness necessary for labor productivity, military readiness, and national security. The movement promoted using calisthenics, sporting activities, weights, and physical apparatus to build strength and muscularity. Advocates brought the movement from Europe to the United States in the 1820s. It spread, aided by published manuals, "muscle magazines," and the popularity of strongmen who lifted huge weights, wrestled animals, and otherwise displayed their strength on the vaudeville and music hall circuits. The initiation of the Modern Olympic Games in 1896 epitomized the patriotic interest in strong male bodies. The new sport of competitive weight lifting was one of the first to be included in the games.

The arrival of a former German circus performer turned strongman at the end of the century changed the concept of the ideal body for American males. Unlike his burly predecessors who provided only displays of functional strength, Eugene Sandow, "The World's Most Perfectly Developed Man," added posed displays of muscular tension. His body, which harked back to ancient Greek statues, had aesthetically pleasing, mesomorphic symmetry and proportion. He promoted his body as a work of art and strength, one that was within reach of every man who was willing to work for it. He became internationally famous and rich by selling manuals, muscle magazines, and equipment in addition to staging demonstrations of strength with his nearly naked body and often posing with scantily clad women in scenes from Greek and Roman mythology.

Tarzan movies, beginning in the early twentieth century, and physique competitions that predated the first Mr. America contest in 1940 and subsequent Mr. Universe and Mr. Olympia competitions reinforced the ideal of mesomorphic muscularity. This ideal survived the decline of vaudeville and the physical culture movement around the time of World War I. A 1921 winner of a physique contest, with the stage name of Charles Atlas, continued to sell the mesomorphic ideal to succeeding generations of young men. His successful advertising formula associated muscularity not only with masculine power, strength, and domination, but also with sexual conquest. Superman and the rest of the superheroes introduced after 1940 linked muscularity to "truth, justice, and the American way." *Hercules* and other "sword and sandal" movies added the attraction of action and adventure to muscularity.

The male ideal of mesomorphic muscularity with its patriotic and militaristic overtones was eclipsed in the second half of the 1960s by the growing opposition to the Vietnam War and the spreading use of illicit drugs. Ectomorphic musicians with shaggy hair, like the Rolling Stones and Bob Dylan, unabashedly put their thin, and sometimes androgynous, bodies on display and became countercultural icons.

The eclipse of muscularity lasted through most of the 1970s. Reflecting the ideology of the times, *The Rocky Horror Show*, a 1973 movie that attracted an enduring cult following, parodied Charles Atlas. The camp Village People broke into the mainstream with their satire "Macho Man" in 1978, shortly after a skinny John Travolta unbuttoned his shirt and danced his way to fame in *Saturday Night Fever*.

Muscularity continued to be valued in the subculture of bodybuilders. They splintered off from weight lifters in the 1920s to concentrate on bigger muscles rather than strength. Ethnographer Alan Klein (1993) says that the subculture's body ideal is driven by narcissism, homophobia, femiphobia, low self-esteem, and insecurity about sexuality and gender. Bodybuilding is their way of asserting control over one aspect of their lives in a period of rapid social change that has left many men feeling socially, politically, and, in some cases, economically powerless. The massively muscular standard is reinforced by competitions, muscle magazines, and other merchandise mainly marketed by the Weider brothers with claims about health, fitness, and sexual potency ("Don't Droop. Put Virility Power into Your Body"). The ideal has grown to freakish proportions with the help of steroids, growth hormones, nutritional supplements, and extreme dietary practices that can endanger physical and mental health. By the 1970s it took the fifty-seven-inch chest and thirty-one-inch waist of Arnold Schwarzenegger to win the Mr. Universe and Mr. Olympia titles.

The declining threat of communism and the return of a more nationalistic conservative political environment with an emphasis on self-reliance in the 1980s provided an opportune time for launching Schwarzenegger's macho, "beef cake" *Conan* and *Terminator* movies along with Sylvester Stallone's *Rocky* and *Rambo* series. Muscular "hard bodies" were back in style, but this time the ideal image was considerably larger, well defined, and harder to attain.

Hard bodies, whether masculine or feminine, have come to symbolize more than just physical strength. They manifest a strong work ethic and strength of character, particularly the presence of self-control and self-discipline. Hard bodies have high status that is independent of other social and economic attributes. Fat, flabbiness, softness, in contrast, is highly stigmatized and connected with laziness and a weak character.

Image Socialization

Technological innovations that inundate society with images of people are another cultural change that influenced the demand for cosmetic surgery. The pervasiveness of these images is a powerful source of socialization about appearance norms. They have helped to narrow the criteria for evaluating appearance.

Early nineteenth-century lithography made it possible to present images in print media. These illustrations, like other forms of art, were not common because their production was time-consuming. Moreover, the images were artistic renderings, not necessarily accurate representations of real people. Awareness of appearance norms depended largely on personal observations of the limited pool of other people in a lo cal area and what was said or written about bodies. In the nineteenth century the message would have included the religious idea that true beauty radiates from internal goodness.

Photography, beginning with the daguerreotype in 1839, revolutionized visual representation. By the 1880s it was possible to reproduce photographs in newspapers and magazines. Editors quickly found that pictures of pretty young women boosted circulation. The photographic beauty contest became a frequent feature in the early twentieth century. The definition of beauty was shifting toward external appearance and away from internal goodness.

Images of beautiful young women in the twentieth century were not confined to the print media and other forms of advertising. They also became a staple of the new motion picture industry, beginning with silent films in 1896. The arrival of television to most homes by the 1950s saturated the public with images of beautiful young women.

The increasingly pervasive images of female beauties did not stop there. Fashion dolls, culminating in Barbie, made an icon out of a caricature of female beauty for young girls to contemplate and internalize. Few can compare themselves favorably to the beautiful women in the media, whose printed pictures are increasingly artificially enhanced. None can measure up to Barbie's cartoonish body. The intensity of socialization about beauty since the middle of the twentieth century explains some of the widespread discontent with personal appearance among women at the end of the century and their increasing rates of cosmetic surgery. Social, psychological, and economic factors that have contributed to the demand for cosmetic surgery are discussed in chapter 2.

The public also has been saturated with visual images of men in the second half of the twentieth century. With the exception of muscle magazines and movies like the *Tarzan, Conan,* and *Rocky* series, the men depicted in general circulation newspapers, magazines, motion pictures, and television have been far more varied in appearance and age than women. In recent years they include men such as entrepreneurs Bill Gates and Ross Perot, actors Danny DeVito and John Lithgow, musicians Mick Jagger and Alice Cooper, and athletes Randy Johnson and Dennis Rodman, who became public figures based on occupational achievements rather than handsomeness. They also include actors Brad Pitt, Tom Cruise, and Denzel Washington, whose celebrity owes something to their visual appeal. Aging does not undermine the careers of professional male beauties as rapidly as it does female beauties. The former, such as Sean Connery and Clint Eastwood, continue to find success and media attention paired with ever younger beautiful women.

The visual diversity of men in the media gives men more opportunities than women to compare themselves favorably and value their own appearance to a greater extent. This gender difference may change. Research reviewed in chapter 2 suggests that appearance is an increasingly important asset for white-collar male workers. Jockey and Calvin Klein demonstrated in the 1980s that muscular male bodies can be as effective in selling merchandise as female bodies. The concept of the "boy toy" came into vogue. Men's health and fitness magazines now advise their growing number of readers on how to achieve the highly desired "great buns" and "buff bodies" with diet, exercise, and cosmetic surgery.

GI Joe, the young boys' toy equivalent of Barbie, although always handsome, did not originally have a cartoon physique. Over time, how-ever, this icon of masculinity has developed seam-splitting muscles, as have other action figures for boys. If scaled to human size, GI Joe's biceps would measure an impossible twenty-six inches. The recent trend toward displaying muscularity is evident in male athletes, mod-els, actors, and the popularity of the World Wrestling Federation and World Championship Wrestling freak show farces. It is associated with an increase in body image problems and steroid abuse in boys and men (Pope et al. 1999). It also is associated with the development of new cosmetic surgery procedures, such as pectoral and calf implants and liposuction techniques to sculpt the rippling "six-pack" abdomi-nal muscles that are characteristic of competitive bodybuilders.

Cosmetic Surgery Defined

Cosmetic surgery is at the cutting edge of a grow-ing commercial sector in medicine. Like other commercial endeavors, cosmetic surgery is a business enterprise aimed at generating profit by selling a product for more than the cost of providing it. Maximiz-ing profit depends both on profit margin and sales volume. As with other commercial ventures, marketing is used to induce sales. It can take the form of paid advertising or unpaid public relations efforts to persuade the public that the product is desirable and worth the ex-pense. The product in this case is surgery and the entrepreneurs are physicians.

Cosmetic surgery differs from noncommercial medical care in several ways. Cosmetic surgery reshapes healthy anatomical structures, the appearance of which falls within the normal range of variation. Cosmetic surgery usually is not covered by health insurance because it is considered an elective procedure without merit for physical health. The optional nature of cosmetic surgery stems from its purpose rather than the techniques used. The goal is to make the patient's appear-ance more closely approximate the contemporary ideal. Cosmetic sur-gery shares techniques and some practitioners with reconstructive surgery, but the goal of reconstructive surgery is different. Reconstruc-tive surgery aims to improve the function and sometimes the appear-ance of abnormal body structures. The abnormalities addressed include those caused by congenital defects, developmental aberrations, trauma, infection, tumors, or disease. Reconstructive surgery usually is not considered elective and is covered by health insurance. Highlighting the distinction, some states mandated coverage of reconstruction of a normal appearance, to the extent possible, when confronted with evidence that some managed care plans denied coverage for babies born with craniofacial defects or for children and adults disfigured by disease, burns, or other traumas on the grounds that the aim of the surgery was only cosmetic (Page 1998).

Reconstructive surgery is part of the much larger noncommercial sector of medicine. Physicians regard this work as a professional service. The demand for reconstructive work and other noncommercial medical care originates in patients' physical needs rather than in marketing campaigns and other sources of cultural pressure. The removal of restrictions against professional advertising in the late 1970s has increased the advertising of all kinds of health care services and blurred the boundary between commercial and noncommercial medicine in some areas of health care. Nevertheless, public advertisements of treatments for burns, hand injuries, or lip and palate clefts are virtually nonexistent. If individual practitioners do any reconstructive patient outreach, it is usually limited to public relations efforts with other kinds of medical specialists, hospitals, and health insurance companies to keep them abreast of what can and should be done for patients with structural abnormalities.

In contrast, cosmetic services are advertised directly to the public in newspapers and magazines and on billboards, radio, television, and Internet websites. Some practitioners employ public relations firms that also place their names with referral services, arrange interviews with reporters, and develop public relations campaigns, such as running public seminars to recruit prospective patients or publishing consumer guidebooks. Most belong to one of several professional associations that publish research journals, sponsor continuing education programs and conferences, operate referral services, and lobby hospitals, legislatures, and insurance companies on behalf of members' occupational interests. These same professional associations also monitor public attitudes toward cosmetic surgery and employ public relations firms to promote both cosmetic surgery and the professional reputation of their members.

Cosmetic Surgery Statistics

Efforts to promote cosmetic surgery have helped create a sunrise industry. Tracking the growth of this industry in the United States is difficult. There are no official government statistics. Most cosmetic procedures take place out of hospital and are absent from the federally monitored hospital discharge data. Medicare, Medicaid, and private health insurance companies provide no data because they categorically deny coverage for procedures designed to modify, rather than restore, a normal appearance. The only available data are from physicians' professional associations that voluntarily collect information from a sample of members to project practice rates for the organization's members. Not all associations collect information. Moreover, there is no legal requirement that a physician who does cosmetic surgery be a member of a professional association, nor that a physician who is a member report personal statistics to the association.

Despite these caveats, there is ample evidence that cosmetic surgery has increased rapidly in recent years. The American Society of Plastic and Reconstructive Surgeons (1999d), an organization representing 97 percent of all physicians certified by the American Board of Plastic Surgery, has used scientific sampling since 1992 to track the cosmetic work of its approximately 5,000 members. It reports that cosmetic surgery procedures by members increased 50 percent between 1996 and 1998 and 153 percent since 1992. Liposuction was the most frequently performed cosmetic procedure by plastic surgeons in 1998, followed by breast augmentation, eyelid surgery, facelift, and chemical face peel. Adding in other procedures such as rhinoplasty (nose), forehead lifts, otoplasty (ear), abdominoplasty (tummy tuck), surgical treatments for baldness, Retin A treatments, and laser skin resurfacing, the organization estimates that members did more than 1 million cosmetic procedures in 1998, only 10 percent less than the estimated number of reconstructive procedures they did. Its sister organization, the American Society for Aesthetic Plastic Surgery, made up of a subset of 1,384 board-certified plastic surgeons who focus mainly on cosmetic work, reports that its members average 320 cosmetic procedures per year (1999).

Plastic surgeons are not the only physicians who offer cosmetic surgery. The American Academy of Facial Plastic and Reconstructive Surgery (1999), an organization mostly made up of otolaryngologists, reports that in 1996 its approximately 2,600 members averaged 241 cosmetic procedures, about two times their reconstructive average. Compared to plastic surgeons, these trained specialists in ear, nose, and throat did more rhinoplasties but far fewer liposuctions and nonfacial procedures such as breast augmentations and abdominoplasties.

Otolaryngologists who expand their cosmetic practice beyond the face and neck are more likely to seek membership in the American

Academy of Cosmetic Surgery, an interdisciplinary association of medical and dental professionals involved in cosmetic surgery. This association also includes general surgeons, dermatologists, ophthalmologists, and oral and maxillofacial surgeons. The organization reports that 57 percent of its 1,100 members do only cosmetic surgery (American Academy of Cosmetic Surgery, 1998, personal communication). The inclusion of dermatologists and practitioners from other backgrounds leads to a different rank order of procedures by members, as compared to plastic surgeons and members of the American Academy of Facial Plastic and Reconstructive Surgery; hair transplants and sclerotherapy (vein treatment) rank in the top five procedures for male patients and sclerotherapy and laser skin resurfacing make the short list for female patients.

The tighter bonds of beauty norms experienced by women as compared to men are reflected in the statistics. The two organizations of board-certified plastic surgeons report that only 9 to 10 percent of members' patients are men. The two other organizations report that 20 percent of members' patients are men. The higher proportion of female patients treated by board-certified plastic surgeons is linked to their higher rates of breast augmentations and breast lifts, compared with otolaryngologists and other specialists in the latter two organizations, who do relatively more rhinoplasties and hair transplants. Although their numbers are growing rapidly, male patients still undergo only a small fraction of all cosmetic surgery procedures because procedures on women are also growing rapidly.

2 | Pretty Pleases

Social, Psychological, and Economic Consequences of Appearance

In 1963 Jimmy Soul spent eleven weeks at the top of the popular music charts with this advice: "If you want to be happy for the rest of you life, never make a pretty woman your wife. So from my personal point of view, get an ugly girl to marry you." The song's popularity derives from its facetious challenge to dominant cultural beliefs about appearance. Attractiveness has long been valued in its own right and associated with other desirable traits. Eighteenth-century Swiss scientist Johann Caspar Lavater claimed that people's behavior could be predicted from their appearances (cited in Finkelstein 1991). The essence of his theory of physiognomy is that virtue produces attractiveness, while vice produces ugliness. Lavater's four-volume treatise connects specific body features to intelligence, morality, and personality and offers one hundred rules for decoding the nuances of appearance.

More than two hundred years later, Levater's lifework is dismissed as fanciful pseudoscience. However, the core assumption that character is immanent in appearance predated him by many centuries and can be traced through Galen and Aristotle to Hippocrates. Moreover, physiognomy continued to flourish long after his death.

Numerous researchers expanded upon Levater's rules. In 1876 Cesare Lombroso used physiognomic theory to predict criminal potential and suggested that high risk individuals—those with small, abnormal, or asymmetrical craniums, low foreheads, large jaws and ears, and crooked or flat noses—be put under surveillance. Others argued that a person could work to change his or her character to achieve a more pleasing appearance. Still others focused more narrowly on the brain and developed the offshoot discipline of phrenology. Phrenologists believed that the size of the bumps and grooves on a person's skull indicated abilities, talents, and character.

Most of the tenets of physiognomy and phrenology seem absurd at the end of the twentieth century. Yet, the research reviewed in this chapter suggests that the core assumption—that character is immanent in appearance—is a persistent belief with social, psychological, and economic consequences. Recognition of these consequences motivates individuals to consider cosmetic surgery. Concern with external appearance has supplanted concern with internal character in the postmodern world. The chapter concludes with a discussion of the social and economic changes that have made concern with appearance a cultural imperative and that support the growing demand for cosmetic surgery.

Social Consequences
Children

Aristotle's belief that "Beauty is a greater recommendation than any letter of introduction" remains as true today as in ancient times. The favorable expectations experienced by attractive people create a more supportive environment that has positive consequences. The rewards of attractiveness begin at birth. Parents are more attentive and affectionate with attractive babies (Langlois 1986; Langlois et al. 1995). Unacquainted child care providers and other adults also attach a favorable stereotype to attractive infants (Casey and Ritter 1996; Karraker and Stern 1990; Ritter et al. 1991; Stephan and Langlois 1984).

Attractive children are similarly favored. Caregivers pay more attention to them than to unattractive children (Hildebrandt and Cannan 1985). Teachers rate them as more intelligent, honest, sociable, popular, and pleasant and are more likely to view them as leaders and less likely to evaluate them negatively for misbehaving (Dion 1972; Kenealy et al. 1988; Lerner et al. 1990; Ritts et al. 1992). Attractive children are also more readily accepted and liked by their peers (Dion 1973; Dion and Berscheid 1974; Kennedy 1990).

To the extent that attractive children are treated as if they are more intelligent, honest, sociable, and natural leaders, they will have more

opportunities to behave accordingly, more opportunities to have con-
firmatory behavior recognized and rewarded, and more opportunities
to internalize this view of themselves. The rewards of attractiveness
have the potential to be cumulative because facial attractiveness from
early childhood through late middle age tends to be stabile, with the
greatest degree of stability during the formative years from childhood
through adolescence (Alley 1993; Zebrowitz, Olson, and Hoffman 1993).

Stability of appearance increases the likelihood of a self-fulfilling
prophecy. Elementary school teachers regard physical attractiveness
as much a determinant of a child's social status as social skills and
an outgoing personality (Maag et al. 1991). By middle school, attractive students have higher grade-point averages and score higher on stan-
dardized achievement tests than unattractive students (Lerner et al.
1990). They also receive more favorable ratings of psychosocial functioning from peers, teachers, and parents (Lerner et al. 1991).

Adults

Attractive adults, like attractive children, enjoy a
favorable stereotype (Dion et al. 1972; Zuckerman et al. 1995). The stereotype reflects the physiognomic maxim that what is beautiful is good.
The content of the stereotype depends on cultural values (Wheeler and
Kim 1997). In Western cultures the stereotype is most consistent for
indexes of social competence, intermediate for measures of social dominance, adjustment, sociability, and intellectual competence, and nearly
nonexistent for moral traits like integrity and concern for others (Eagly
et al. 1991). The stereotype is the same for men and women, except
attractive women also are expected to have more sexual warmth (Feingold 1990).

Stereotypic expectations based on appearance merely create the
possibility of a self-fulfilling prophecy; they do not predestine it. Other
ascribed characteristics such as race, sex, and age carry their own stereotypes. Individual experiences such as childhood nurturing, opportunities to acquire and express skills, and feedback also contribute to
achieved competencies. Consequently, the correlations between objective measures of physical attractiveness and actual social and intellectual competence are small (Feingold 1992). Nevertheless, the
relationships are usually positive and statistically significant, supporting the existence of a self-fulfilling prophecy. Some of the most
persuasive evidence that the attractiveness stereotype has social consequences are the findings that attractive adults are less lonely, less

socially anxious, more popular, more socially skilled, date more, and are more sexually experienced than unattractive people.

There is a wealth of evidence that attractiveness is an important asset for dating, although there is a strong gender difference in its degree of importance (Feingold 1990). Women also are influenced by a man's socioeconomic status; they are four times more likely to respond to a personal advertisement of an average-looking professional than a handsome cabdriver (Goode 1996). In contrast, men are nearly three times more likely to respond to a personal advertisement of a woman who claims a high degree of physical attractiveness than one who claims only average attractiveness, even when the latter advertises significantly higher socioeconomic status. The strong male preference for attractiveness is independent of sexual orientation (Hatala and Prehodka 1996; Smith et al. 1990).

There is overwhelming evidence that attractiveness influences women's romantic experiences (Jackson 1992). Very attractive women date more, fall in love more, and have more sexual experiences than women of average or less attractiveness. Although women are significantly less likely to request attractiveness in a prospective partner and are more likely to seek a compatible personality than men, they are not immune to the allure of attractiveness, as the high correlation between the number of sexual partners and the attractiveness of university men demonstrates (Bogaert and Fisher 1995).

Both women and men underestimate the influence of physical attractiveness on their initial assessment of potential dates and mates (Sprecher 1989). Physical attractiveness also influences perceptions of sexual advances, at least in hypothetical situations. Both young women and young men are less likely to perceive sexual advances from members of the opposite sex as sexual harassment if the initiator is described as attractive and the level of coercion reported is not high (Carter et al. 1996; Struckman-Johnson and Struckman-Johnson 1994). When the level of coercion involved is high, young men are still less likely to view the incident as sexual harassment if the woman initiating the sexual advance is said to be attractive.

As with dating, physical attractiveness plays a significant role in marital prospects and again its impact is greater for women than men (Hatfield and Sprecher 1995). Men's preference may reflect more than personal taste because men are regarded as more sociable, friendly, and self-confident by others when they are in the company of attractive women (Sigall and Landy 1973). As a result, attractive women have a higher value in the marriage "market." Not only are highly attractive women more likely to marry than less attractive women, they also are more likely to marry men of higher socioeconomic status (Udry and Eckland 1984). Although the marital prospects of men do not appear to be as dependent upon attractiveness as they are for women, attractive men are more likely to succeed in marrying attractive women. When couples are mismatched on physical attractiveness, they typically involve a more attractive woman married to a less attractive, but prosperous, man.

A comparison of dating and married couples suggests that most couples first assort on physical traits, although they are likely to marry only if they also are similar on psychological traits (Keller and Young 1996). Physical attractiveness continues to exert a significant impact after marriage. More attractive people report more satisfaction with their marriages. Perceived declines in the physical attractiveness of wives diminish husbands' interest in sexual relations and increase the likelihood of reporting sexual problems in their marriages (Margolin and White 1987). This effect, unique to husbands, is not reduced by age, marital duration, or economic well-being.

Seeking a deeper meaning to the finding that "pretty pleases" in dating and mating, researchers have offered evolutionary explanations. Although some aspects of attractiveness, such as preferences for body weight and the various types of body modifications, discussed in chapter 1, are clearly culturally constructed, others may be biologically constructed and connected to health and reproductive potential.

There is a remarkably high level of consensus about a person's degree of attractiveness (Patzer 1985; Zebrowitz, Montepare, and Lee 1993) and some fundamental attributes are valued across cultures (Cunningham et al. 1995). Like other species, humans favor average facial features and overall facial and body symmetry, characteristics that researchers argue signal a reduced likelihood of harmful genetic mutations, external developmental traumas, and the residual effects of disease, along with a greater likelihood of high genetic diversity that would provide greater disease resistance (Langlois and Roggman 1990; Thornhill and Gangestad 1993). A test of this "fitness" hypothesis reveals that ratings of facial attractiveness are highly correlated with observers' ratings of perceived health, but not actual health (Kalick et al. 1998). The health of very attractive people is overestimated and the health of very unattractive people is underestimated. In other words, we are more accurate in assessing the health of average-looking individuals. Apparently the stereotype associated with appearance can be blinding at either extreme.

While average faces are judged to be attractive, the faces judged to be exceptionally attractive are not necessarily average, nor are they randomly different from average. Instead, blindingly beautiful faces, while still symmetrical, have exaggerated sex-linked features (Perrett et al. 1994). The ideal male has a strong jaw and prominent eyebrow ridges, characteristics associated with male sex hormones and strength. In contrast, the ideal female has a higher than average forehead, smaller nose, fuller lips, and a smaller jaw, characteristics associated with youth and potential fertility (Johnson and Franklin 1993).

The ideal female body also reflects fertility potential. However, unlike the ideal female face, the prized American female body at the end of the twentieth century is much thinner than the population average. The same is true for the ideal male body. The average weights of both sexes have increased considerably over time (Hill and Peters 1998). Despite this increase, the female ideal, as embodied in Miss America winners and *Playboy* centerfolds, has become thinner, except in the bust area. There has been no corresponding thinning of male models in *Esquire* and *GQ* magazines, nor, as social critics point out, a corresponding epidemic of anorexia and bulimia among young men (Petrie et al. 1996).

Although ideal female body weight appears to be culturally variant and highly fluid over time, the ideal shape, as measured by the waist-to-hip ratio, is highly consistent, even among the ever-leaner Miss America winners and *Playboy* centerfolds (Singh 1993). Men of all ages and from diverse cultures prefer women with a narrow waist relative to hip width, a shape characteristic of women in their fertile years (Furnham et al. 1997). The waist-to-hip ratio appears to be a more important determinant of male assessment of female attractiveness than breast size or weight (Singh 1994, 1995). The waist-to-hip ratio also is an important determinant of female assessment of male attractiveness (Singh 1995), as is height, another cue to puberty and physical strength.

Research findings to date can be interpreted to support the sociobiological contention that evolutionary forces play at least a partial role in determining why pretty pleases in dating and mating. Women who display youth and fecundity are more desirable because of their higher reproductive value. In contrast, a man's fertile period is not as dependent on youth as is a woman's. Therefore, health and strength are more salient cues to a man's reproductive value than youth. Why pretty pleases in other interpersonal relationships—between parents and children, teachers and children, and between peers—is more difficult to attribute directly to underlying evolutionary forces. It may be a halo effect, an overgeneralization, of an internalized preference for attractiveness, a preference that has been observed in infants before an awareness of cultural stereotypes and the social power associated with attractiveness could be learned (Langlois et al. 1991). Nevertheless, cultural forces also play a role in shaping preferences for some aspects of appearance, as the examples in chapter 1 demonstrate. Whether biological or cultural in origin, the consequences of preferences for particular appearance attributes are substantial and extend well beyond the impact on dating and mating.

Experiments show that less attractive people in need of assistance, such as in a stalled car or after a fall, receive fewer offers of help from strangers than more attractive people (Patzer 1985, 70–78). Even health care professionals are influenced by the appearance of patients (Zebrowitz 1997, 157–158). Physicians give more nonverbal attention and show more courtesy to attractive patients than to unattractive patients. Being unattractive does have some advantages; physicians are more likely to take the pain complaints of such patients seriously, perhaps because they unconsciously associate unattractiveness with illness.

The appearance stereotype also may influence judicial outcomes (Zebrowitz 1997, 154–156). Mock juries are less likely to convict attractive defendants and are more likely to give them lenient sentences unless their transgressions take advantage of their appearances. Attractive plaintiffs also are favored in actual judicial rulings. Psychologists have long suspected that the significant differences in treatment elicited by appearance influence personality development and mental health.

Psychological Consequences

Extroversion, conscientiousness, agreeableness, culture (artistic sensibility), and emotional stability are fundamental components of personality (Zebrowitz 1997, 42–46). These traits vary considerably between individuals and are highly stable by young adulthood. Extroversion, a composite measure of how open, talkative, sociable, and adventurous a person is, shows a moderate-to-strong association with facial appearance. People perceived to be more extroverted by strangers are more likely to claim to be extroverted, exhibit more extroverted behaviors, and be judged by their friends to be extroverted.

None of the other "big five" personality traits show as strong an association with perceived appearance as extroversion. There is only a small-to-moderate association between a conscientious appearance and a conscientious personality. There is little consensus about the appearance of agreeableness, culture, and emotional stability and, consequently, no association between perceived appearance and these personality traits.

Psychological traits expected to have evolutionary implications show stronger associations with appearance. These include sexual availability, social dominance, intelligence, and honesty. Sexual availability (measured by sexual permissiveness and sexual activity) shows the strongest relationship with perceived appearance. We can more accurately identify available sexual partners than extroverted or conscientious individuals. We also can recognize leadership traits moderately well from appearance alone. The findings for intelligence also suggest a moderate degree of accuracy for judgements based on appearance. The findings on honesty, however, point to the complexity of the relationship between appearance and personality traits.

The halo effect of attractiveness includes the assumption that attractive people are more likely to be honest (Zebrowitz et al. 1996). However, sociobiological theory suggests that it would be adaptive to conceal one's dishonesty. Perhaps for this reason appearance is an unreliable cue for honesty. This finding does not mean that appearance has no affect on the development of an honest personality. Men who looked more honest and attractive as children scored higher on honesty in their thirties and fifties than others. The effect is largest for those whose appearance was stable over time. Such findings support the self-fulfilling prophecy hypothesis, but only for men. Women show an "artifice" effect. Those who scored higher on dishonesty early in life developed more honest-looking and more attractive appearances in later life, making them indistinguishable from women with honest personalities. Women inclined to dishonesty may have few scruples about improving their appearances to reap the considerable social rewards given to attractive women.

When it comes to appearances, the stakes for both men and women include psychological well-being in addition to social rewards. Being attractive in the eyes of others is conducive to mental health (Umberson and Hughes 1987). Higher levels of attractiveness are associated with higher levels of life satisfaction, lower levels of perceived stress, a greater sense of personal competence, and a more positive and balanced affect—that is, how we feel about our everyday experiences. The relationships persist when other strong predictors of well-being, including age, race, education, income, occupational prestige, and employment status, are taken into account. Attractiveness is most strongly associated with sense of personal competence. In general, the more attractive a person is, the more competent and in control of their lives they feel, affirming the attractiveness stereotype. The strength of the other relationships indicates that appearance has a greater impact on everyday experiences than overall life satisfaction or perceived stress, although it affects these as well. Attractive people are more satisfied with their lives, perceive less stress, and feel more positive and happy about everyday events.

Despite the association between objective measures of attractiveness and psychological well-being, being considered attractive has only a small positive association with the global psychological construct of self-esteem (Jackson 1992, 130–132). Self-concept is highly subjective and multifaceted. Objective measures of attractiveness are only weakly correlated with self-evaluation. Factors other than a mirror influence our self-perceptions. Self-ratings of attractiveness show stronger, though still modest, relationships with self-esteem. Appearance may be central to some people's sense of self-worth and tangential to others (Sarwer et al. 1998).

The importance placed on specific appearance features varies widely. In extreme psychopathological cases individuals engage in obsessive preoccupation with some body part, repeatedly checking, examining, or trying to hide an imagined or slight flaw. As a result, the associations between self-ratings of attractiveness and self-esteem are not as strong as one might expect if self-esteem were mainly a consequence of an overall favorable assessment of personal appearance, rather than one of many precursors to it. There is evidence of the latter. Global self-orientations such as self-esteem and social desirability account for some of the observed association between subjective attractiveness and personality attributes (Longo and Ashmore 1995). Gender, another global self-orientation, also affects self-ratings of attractiveness and self-esteem; females score significantly lower than males on both measures (Nell and Ashton 1996). There is a growing consensus that body image, including how one thinks and feels about one's body, is shaped by cultural influences (Sarwer et al. 1998).

Dissatisfaction with personal appearance is widespread. Approximately one-half of all women and one-fourth of all men in the United States dislike at least some aspect of their looks (Cash 1997). The greater dissatisfaction of women cannot be attributed to objective sex differences in physical attractiveness because strangers invariably rate women as a group better looking than men. Instead, the gender difference reflects more intense social pressures on women to be attractive in American society. Today that means being symmetrical and thin with a low waist-to-hip ratio and average or exaggerated sex-linked features. The increasing gender difference in satisfaction with appearance over the last fifty years supports the widely held belief that cultural pressures to be attractive have intensified, especially for women (Feingold and Mazzella 1998). Part of this change may stem from the recognition that appearance has concrete economic as well as social consequences.

Economic Consequences

The stereotypic belief that attractiveness is a sign of competency extends from children to adults, despite no evidence of such a general association among adults (Jackson et al. 1995). The stereotype is stronger for men than women, who are subjected to gender bias as well. Attractive politicians are assumed to be more competent (Lewis and Bierly 1990). Attractive professors are assumed to be better teachers (Romano and Bordiere 1989). Attractive counselors are assumed to be more helpful (Green et al. 1986). Attractive salespersons are assumed to be more effective (Reingen and Kernan 1993). There is additional evidence that in at least some occupations these expectations create a self-fulfilling prophecy. More attractive salespeople tend to be more effective (DeShields et al. 1996), and people report feeling more comfortable disclosing problems to a more attractive female therapist than a less attractive one (Harris and Busby 1998). Whether attractive male therapists are similarly advantaged remains to be determined. Nevertheless, there is ample additional evidence that attractiveness is an asset in the workplace.

Perceptions of competency based on appearance influence hiring decisions. Favoritism toward attractive applicants is strongest for jobs that involve interpersonal contact (Collins and Zebrowitz 1995). For example, professional recruiters' ratings of MBA job candidates at a prestigious Ivy League business school indicate that they are more influenced by a job candidate's physical attractiveness than objective qualifications (Rynes and Gerhart 1990). Managers' ratings of hypothetical managerial job candidates similarly show strong evidence of an attractiveness bias (Marlowe et al. 1996). The ratings reveal an additional persistent gender bias. More experienced managers are somewhat less prejudiced; however, all discriminate against less attractive women applicants, regardless of the qualifications listed on their résumés.

Appearance has an impact on performance evaluations and promotion decisions. Although earlier studies reported that attractive women were penalized when seeking or holding managerial or other traditionally male jobs, more recent research indicates that attractive women now receive higher overall evaluations, regardless of job type, as do attractive men (Drogosz and Levy 1996). The bias is less when older personnel professionals make recommendations for promotion to more senior positions, although it is still significant (Morrow et al. 1990).

Good looks also pay off in higher earnings. Attractive workers have more prestigious jobs and earn more money than less attractive workers when race, age, education, and other relevant variables are taken into account (Umberson and Hughes 1987). The bias is consistent across all job skill levels, although the degree of difference is greatest for low- and moderate-skill occupations. In general, unattractive people earn 5 to 10 percent less than average-looking people. Very attractive people earn approximately 5 percent more, after credentials, occupation, and age are taken into consideration (Hamermesh and Biddle 1994). Only a small portion of the observed wage difference can be explained by the tendency for very attractive people to gravitate to occupations where appearance is more salient.

The "plainness penalty" and the "beauty bonus" exist in almost all occupations and the effects are cumulative. Graduates of a prestigious law school whose matriculation photographs ranked in the top third on attractiveness earned 9 percent more on average five years after graduation than those whose photographs ranked in the bottom third (Biddle and Hamermesh 1998). Fifteen years after graduation the earnings difference had grown to 13 percent. In general, attractive law school graduates gravitated to the private sector where wages are higher than in the public sector. However, public sector jobs are not impervious to the impact of beauty; attractive graduates of military service academies have more successful careers (Dickey-Bryant et al. 1986). A study of MBA graduates reports similar findings on the cumulative impact of facial attractiveness on salary growth (Frieze et al. 1991). This research reveals that height and weight additionally influence salaries.

Employers are willing to pay a premium for tall workers. They also discriminate against fat workers in some positions. Tall full-time workers earn approximately 4 to 6 percent more than those shorter than average (Loh 1993). The advantage of being tall is greater for men than women. The effect of body weight on wages varies, depending on the population examined. Weight appears to have no impact on the starting wages of young adults (Umberson and Hughes 1987). Obese men, however, have about 5 percent less wage growth over a three year period than non-obese men. Obese women in higher status professional, technical, and management positions are similarly penalized (Haskins 1990).

Social Change and the Demand for Cosmetic Surgery

The growing demand for cosmetic surgery is a product of the larger culture. The research reviewed in this chapter leaves little doubt that attractiveness has real social, psychological, and economic value in America. Like race, ethnicity, gender, and age, appearance confers a status. Unlike these other master statuses, appearance can be enhanced through the use of makeup, hairstyle, and various forms of adornment and body modifications, such as those mentioned in chapter 1. Individuals who turn to cosmetic surgery to carve a more attractive appearance, like the Padaung women who elongate their necks with rings and the Africans who decorate their bodies with elaborate patterns of scars, are making a rational response to prevailing cultural values that reward those considered more attractive and penalize those considered less attractive. Cosmetic surgery can be a means of achieving upward social mobility in such a culture.

The standards used to evaluate attractiveness in a particular culture have both sociobiological and cultural components. Although not yet well-understood, the former would be constant across cultures and time. The latter, in contrast, vary. Age is valued in traditional agricultural societies where children abound and experienced elders are rare. Light skin is valued in racially diverse societies where northern Europeans occupy positions of power. Fat is valued in cultures were food is scarce and weight is an indicator of socioeconomic status. Thinness is valued in consumer societies where obesity is common and weight control is a cue to internal discipline amid abundance. As these examples demonstrate, the cultural components of attractiveness are fluid and reflect the larger political economy and emerging social structure.

There have been numerous changes in American society over the twentieth century, changes that have made an attractive appearance more valuable and turned cosmetic surgery into a sunrise industry in recent decades. One of the most obvious has been the change in the occupational structure of the economy. As employment in agriculture and factory jobs declined, employment in service sector, professional, and management jobs expanded. The tasks of most white-collar jobs involve far more interpersonal contacts than the tasks of blue-collar jobs. The more interpersonal contacts a worker has, the more opportunities he or she has to experience discrimination or favoritism based on appearance. Decreased white-collar job stability in the new "right-sized" corporate culture adds to appearance anxiety in postindustrial economies and explains some of the motivation behind the decision to undergo cosmetic surgery.

Middle- and upper-class women joined the paid labor force at the same time the occupational structure was changing. This added role puts women in the public domain where stereotypes about gender, age, and appearance persist. Aging women are particularly vulnerable to discrimination in the workplace, and some regard cosmetic surgery as a tool to assert some control over their visible signs of aging and to diminish the stigma. Their wages, together with financing programs, provide the discretionary income needed to pay the costs, which averaged almost $5,000 in physician fees for a facelift in 1998 (American Society of Plastic and Reconstructive Surgeons 1999a). Eyelid surgery would add about $3,000 in physician fees, and a forehead lift would add another $2,500 for the average patient. Other potential costs include use of a surgical facility, an anesthesiologist, nurses, and medicines.

The importance of appearance for dating and mating, particularly for women, points to another domain where stereotypes about gender, age, and appearance persist. Radical changes have occurred in this private domain in the last three decades, exposing men and women to more years of dating and dating at older ages. Median age of marriage for both has increased four years (Bureau of the Census 1999). As a result, nearly one in three men and one in five women in their early thirties have not yet married. More than half of those who marry become single again after a divorce. Single women who want a husband face an increasingly tight "marriage market" as they age; this is exacerbated by higher male mortality and cultural norms that expect men to marry younger women, with the age gap increasing at older ages. Physical attractiveness, whether endowed by nature or enhanced by choice, is a valuable currency for women in this marketplace.

Although the social pressures for an attractive, youthful appearance are stronger for women than men, men have not escaped the repercussions. Surgical treatments for male-patterned baldness averaged about $3,000 to $4,000 in physician fees in 1998. Men accounted for 45 percent of board-certified plastic surgeons' ear surgeries ($2,500) and approximately one-fourth of their chin augmentations ($1,600), cheek implants ($2,100), and nose operations (American Society of Plastic and Reconstructive Surgeons 1999a, 1999c). Changing the appearance of a nose averaged between $3,000 and $3,400, depending on the procedure used. The number of men seeking other types of cosmetic surgery also is increasing. Men's facelifts doubled between 1992 and 1998. The number of liposuction procedures (about $2,000 to $4,000 per site) more than tripled and was the most common male procedure done by board-certified plastic surgeons, followed by eyelid surgery.

The number of liposuctions on women increased almost as much as on men over the same period. Breast augmentations, however, increased the most, 306 percent since 1992 when the FDA moratorium went into effect and media coverage raised questions about health risks. Physicians have since switched to saline implants. Breast reconstruction ($3,000 to $9,500) increased 135 percent and breast reduction ($5,500) increased 77 percent over the same period. As a result, in spite of large increases in many kinds of cosmetic surgery on men, men only accounted for 9 percent of board-certified plastic surgeons' work in 1998.

The gender gap in cosmetic surgery may shrink. More physicians now offer cosmetic procedures to enhance masculine body features, including controversial operations to make a penis appear longer and thicker when not erect. New liposuction techniques can sculpt abdominal muscle definition, which, along with pectoral and calf implants, can help men achieve the powerful, disciplined, bodybuilder physique that has become the ideal at the close of the twentieth century.

Attitudes toward cosmetic surgery are increasingly favorable. A 1997 national survey sponsored by the American Society of Plastic and Reconstructive Surgeons (1998a) reveals that 47 percent of women and 34 percent of men say that they have more favorable attitudes toward cosmetic surgery now than ten years ago. Sixty-eight percent of women and 58 percent of men approve of cosmetic surgery for themselves or for others. Most of the rest are undecided about it; only 11 percent of women and 14 percent of men disapprove of it. Approval is highest among middle-aged respondents. More than one-fifth of forty-five- to fifty-four-year-old respondents report that they either have undergone cosmetic surgery or think they will at some point in their lives. As would be expected from the literature reviewed in this chapter, women are more than twice as likely as men to have had or expect to have cosmetic surgery (19 versus 7 percent). These women and their male counterparts want to be as attractive as possible because pretty pleases in personal relationships and in the workplace. The next chapter traces the evolution of the surgical techniques that make such changes possible.

3

Technological Imperialism

The Emergence of Cosmetic Surgery

The research reviewed in chapter 2 suggests that appearance is a master status in modern American society, equivalent to age, gender, social class, and race. An attractive appearance confers measurable social and economic rewards because an attractive exterior is assumed to be associated with valued inner qualities such as intelligence, kindness, and self-control. In contrast, other research reveals that an "impaired" appearance, one that is deviant because of obvious deformities, is stigmatized (Goffman 1967; Beuf 1990). Individuals with impaired appearances tend to be objectified in terms of their appearance flaw, negatively stereotyped, and shunned to varying degrees. From Richard III and Rumpelstiltskin to Frankenstein and the Joker, an impaired appearance is associated with greed, evil, and menace. While the high value accorded beauty may be a modern development amplified by the impact of visual forms of mass media, establishing a social distance from individuals with a deviant appearance may be primordial.

The birth of an infant with a congenital deformity in premodern societies was believed to portend disaster. The oldest surviving written works about congenital deformities are the "omen-texts" of Assurbanipal, King of Assyria, more than six hundred years BCE (Stricker et al. 1990). Like disease, congenital malformations have been viewed as divine punishment for sin, the work of witches, or the result of disturbing events seen by a mother during her pregnancy. Deformed babies often were discarded. The Spartans threw them from the Taygetus Mountain and the Romans drowned them in the Tiber. In later societies, some who survived with anomalies were displayed as freakish human curiosities. Most of the rest lived in the shadows of society, hidden by families or begging for charity.

A normal body at birth provides no protection against the subsequent distorting effects and associated stigma of developmental disorders such as acromegaly or trauma and disease. Since ancient times some individuals with noticeable deformities, particularly facial deformities that cannot be covered by clothing, have sought surgery to try to attain an appearance that falls within the normal range of variation, an appearance that would free them from the burden of social stigma. This chapter begins with a brief history of efforts to reconstruct a more normal appearance for the disfigured, efforts that led to the modern medical specialty of plastic surgery. The evolution of reconstructive surgery provided the techniques that some physicians began to use to enhance the appearance of normal-looking individuals. As demand for surgical enhancement of normal appearances increased, cosmetic techniques multiplied. The chapter describes the most common cosmetic procedures and concludes with a discussion of the ethical dilemmas such cosmetic procedures present for medicine.

The History of Reconstructive Surgery

Plastic surgery dates back to ancient times when deformities were sometimes caused by punishment as well as by congenital anomalies, accidents, and the ravages of war and disease. Accidents, war, and diseases such as syphilis have always mutilated bodies, but noses, ears, eyelids, fingers, hands, and feet also were amputated as retribution in some societies. Adulterous wives, thieves, and captured soldiers were most likely to be subjected to these mortifications and resulting stigma.

Ancient Times

The *Sushruta Samhita,* written in approximately 600 BCE and based on the Hindu hymn *Rig Veda*, which originated some nine hundred years before, contains the oldest known written account of surgical reconstruction of noses and ear lobes (Brown 1986). The procedures were done by a few families in the lowly Hindu castes of potters and bricklayers long before the development of anesthesia, asepsis, and antibiotics. To rebuild a nose they partially sliced a patch of skin from the cheek to form an attached flap, scarified it with a knife, and swung it over the "refreshed" nose wound. They finished the procedure by inserting small pipes to maintain nostril openings and shaping the tissue with a bandage to resemble a nose. Ear lobes were similarly reconstructed using adjacent flaps of skin (Rogers 1988).

By the mid-fifteenth century Hindu practitioners had substituted forehead flaps. This sophisticated procedure was introduced to the Western world in a 1794 edition of *The Gentlemen's Magazine.* Twenty years later, still long before anesthesia, blood transfusion, asepsis, and antibiotics, a British physician reported using the "Indian method." Rogers (1988) regards this operation as the impetus for the development of every plastic surgery procedure since then.

There were, however, other important developments in the evolution of plastic surgery. In the only complete medical text to survive from antiquity, *De medicina,* Cornelius Celsus (25 BCE–50 CE) described the use of double-pedicled advancement flaps of skin to close gapping wounds and the excision of excess skin from "relaxed eyelids." He even recommended using a woman's hair as thread for fine sutures on the face. Undoubtedly others continued at least simple reconstructions over the centuries. Paulus Aegineta, a Greek physician practicing in seventh-century Alexandria, described many of the same techniques as Celsus as well as treatments for jaw and nasal fractures. In the fifteenth century Serafeddin Sabuncuoglu authored the first known illustrated surgical textbook in the Turkish-Islamic literature, in which he described techniques for eyelid problems, facial fractures, and reduction mammoplasty for male gynecomastia (Dogan et al. 1997). However, the medieval Catholic Church opposed such operations on the grounds they interfered with Divine Will. As a result, few European records of reconstructive surgery exist before the Renaissance.

Renaissance

A fourteenth-century Flemish surgeon, Jehan Yperman, described how to repair harelips, as did sixteenth-century French Huguenot Ambroise Paré, widely regarded as the most skilled surgeon of the Renaissance (Rogers 1988). Paré also described many eyelid repairs, but he apparently did not appreciate the reconstructive surgical techniques used in the south of Italy, techniques that laid the cornerstone of plastic surgery in the Western world.

Branca, a fifteenth-century barber-surgeon from Catania in Sicily, reconstructed noses using cheek flaps (Patterson 1977, 3–14). His son Antonio substituted a partially severed upper arm skin flap for a forehead flap to avoid additional scarring on the face. He also used upper arm flaps to reconstruct lips and ears. How many others, if any, engaged in reconstructive surgery in fifteenth-century Europe are unknown; secrecy surrounded such operations. The Vianeo family (also know as Vianeus and Bojanis) reconstructed facial features from the early to mid-sixteenth century in nearby Calabria. They, too, left no personal records, although Leonardo Fioravanti, a trained surgeon from Bologna, published a description of their procedure in 1570 (Santoni-Rugiu and Mazzola 1997).

The "Italian method" was grueling. Patients had to endure numerous operative procedures without anesthesia. They also suffered the pain of having their arms immobilized over their heads for several weeks to allow the flap of skin cut from the upper arms to remain attached to the arm's blood supply while the edges of the flap, sutured over the nasal area, had time to adhere. Afterwards the arm connection was severed and the flap was sewn above the lip. The new nose was shaped with nostril openings. Although there is no evidence that Fioravanti attempted a nose reconstruction, his account provided the information necessary for others who were willing to try such a complicated, lengthy, and painful procedure.

The challenge was taken up by Gaspare Tagliacozzi (also known as Taliacotius, Taliacott, Tagliacozza, and Tag). He was a medical student at the University of Bologna when Fioravanti was accepted into the famous Collegio de' Dottori of Bologna. Tagliacozzi did lip and ear reconstructions, as well as noses, using arm skin flaps. Two years before his death in 1599 and after more than a decade of reconstructions with attached flaps, he published the first book devoted to plastic surgery, De Curtorum Chirurgia per Insitionem. In it he clarified his purpose: "We bring back, refashion and restore to wholeness the features which nature gave but chance destroyed, not that they may charm the eye but that they may be an advantage to the living soul . . . the end for which the physician is working is that the features should fulfill their offices according to nature's decree" (qtd. in Brown 1986).

Tagliacozzi's forthright acknowledgment of his work made him both famous and infamous. On the one hand, he was memorialized by colleagues and students in statues erected at the University of Bologna and the University of Padua after he died. On the other hand, his remains were rumored to have been exhumed from a church

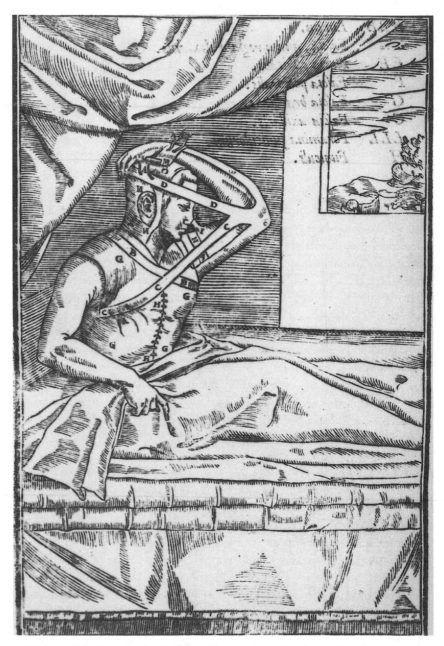

Figure 3.1. Nose reconstruction illustrated in *De Curtorum Chirurgia per Insitionem*, published in Venice by Gaspare Tagliacozzi in 1597. *Courtesy of the National Library of Medicine, Images from the History of Medicine.*

cemetery and reburied in unconsecrated ground after reports that a disembodied voice cried out at night, "Taliacotius is damned" (Updegraff 1938). All copies of his book were ordered destroyed when the church tried to halt the encroachment on its authority by medical science. Paré and other highly regarded physicians maligned him. They turned to prosthetics to help the maimed (Ring 1991).

Even before Tagliacozzi's death, the boundary between reconstructive surgery fact and myth was blurred. Others claimed that detached skin from the buttocks or from another person could be used in reconstructions, although there is no record that any of them tried such procedures. Tagliacozzi refuted these ideas in his textbook. Nevertheless, the myths persisted and were embellished over time. In 1710 the British *Tatler* claimed that "Tag" had reconstructed the noses of three Spaniards with skin from another man's buttocks. When the skin donor was subsequently beaten, the new noses reportedly swelled in pain, forcing the Spaniards to protect their donor, who was said to have "led them by the nose." The author also claimed that the incision sites on the donor itched when one of the reconstructed noses smelled pepper or other strong spice. In another case a reconstructed nose supposedly fell off when the skin donor died. Such foolishness took its toll. Updegraff concluded that "in the seventeenth and eighteenth centuries, the art of facial restoration was in such disrepute as to become almost forgotten" (1938, 650).

Although Tagliacozzi claimed to have improved earlier reconstructive techniques, German surgeon Eduard Zeis provided persuasive evidence to the contrary in his exhaustive 1863 history of what he had called "plastic surgery" in his earlier 1838 book (Patterson 1977, 7–11). Nevertheless, Zeis acknowledged that Tagliacozzi, who today is regarded by most physicians as the father of plastic surgery, carried out a number of these operations and provided more detailed accounts of the techniques, including illustrations, than had anyone previously. Zeis found credible evidence of only four other practitioners in Europe who tried to reconstruct noses at the same time as Tagliacozzi or soon after him. However, he found no evidence of any European doing nose reconstruction in the second half of the seventeenth century.

Nineteenth-Century Reemergence

Reconstructive surgery reemerged in the West after the 1794 article on Indian nose reconstruction in *The Gentlemen's Magazine*. The time had come again for surgeons to explore the possibilities. A British surgeon, Joseph Carpue, successfully reconstructed two noses in 1814 and 1815 using the Indian technique (Patterson 1977, 90–121). Carl Ferdinand von Graefe, a professor of surgery in Berlin, began using the Italian technique in 1816. His first procedure took eleven months to complete. As he gained experience, he gradually developed a German method that combined the first three of Tagliacozzi's six surgical steps to make a nose. Von Graefe's approach to what he called "Rhinoplastik" greatly shortened the time, although the necessity of toughening the skin added to the patient's discomfort. Few other surgeons followed von Graefe's lead. Despite the forehead scar, they found the simpler Indian method more reliable and wanted to spare patients the agony of an arm immobilized over the head for several weeks.

Although other surgeons did not follow von Graefe's approach to nose reconstruction, he still is considered the founder of modern plastic surgery by most because of the breadth of his reconstructive work (Rogers 1988). He successfully reconstructed the lower eyelid of a young girl in 1809 by rotating skin from the cheek. He successfully closed a soft cleft palate in 1816, an astonishing feat at the time, and reconstructed a lower eyelid, cheek, and adjacent nasal region using a forehead flap in 1821. He also tried to use detached skin grafts for repairs, but, like other contemporaries who experimented with them, his efforts were not successful.

One of von Graefe's contemporaries, Johann Friedrich Dieffenbach, achieved considerable success with the Indian method of nose reconstruction. He improved the procedure in a number of ways, including reducing blood congestion with leeches and reducing the compression of vessels in the pedicle (skin bridge) of the forehead flap by insetting the pedicle, rather than laying it over the intact skin between the eyes (Patterson 1977, 94–99). He simplified von Graefe's technique for closing soft cleft palates and was the first to operate on a hard cleft palate using bone flaps. He also improved techniques to reconstruct the area around the eyes. Dieffenbach published descriptions of his innovations in his highly esteemed book, *Die operative Chirurgie* (1845). He is most famous, however, for nose reconstruction in severely mutilated faces. When replacement using forehead skin was not feasible, he constructed a complete "nose" on the patient's arm. The process took about six weeks. Then he transferred it to the nose area, immobilizing the patient's arm in a manner similar to the Italian method, but only for about two weeks.

Z-plasty emerged in the middle of the nineteenth century and became one of the fundamental plastic techniques in the eye region in the second half of that century (Rogers 1988). More surgeons began to experiment with flaps for reconstruction. Their efforts were enhanced by the introduction of anesthesia and antiseptic techniques in the latter part of the nineteenth century. The stage was set for successful detached skin grafts.

Jacques Reverdin, a Swiss surgeon working in Paris, usually is credited with the first successful detached skin grafts in 1869, although there are a few earlier reports of successful operations. He, however, attributed the spread of grafting to the earlier work of George Pollock in London (Freshwater 1984). There is no ambiguity about the subsequent developments; Reverdin's small, pinch-like, free grafts of skin hastened the healing of granulating wounds and led the way to successful larger, thicker, detached skin grafts and split-thickness grafts that contained all of the epidermis but only a thin layer of dermis. By the 1890s most of skin grafting techniques used one hundred years later had been described by nineteenth-century surgical pioneers, although such operations were rare (Rogers 1988).

Gaining Respect in World War I

Trench warfare in World War I blew away jaws, lips, noses, cheek bones, and eyes. Airplane crashes added more injuries. Historian Elizabeth Haiken (1994) points out that the horrifying facial wounds were immediately recognized not only as a surgical problem, but also as a social problem. The unprecedented nature of the injuries challenged the most highly trained medical and dental surgeons of the day to push past the previous boundaries of reconstructive surgery. As they sought to restore function, they also tried to create an appearance that would allow a veteran to return to his family and his work, thereby retaining his sense of independent manhood. Most of the injured were willing to undergo virtually any ordeal, no matter how painful, to attain this goal. Grafts and flaps of all types were used by the men who would become the founders of the new specialty of plastic surgery after the war.

Harold Delf Gillies, a New Zealand otolaryngologist (a specialist in ear, nose, and throat problems), directed a reconstructive medical unit in England. He began to sew together the parallel sides of the skin bridges used to supply flaps with blood. These "tubed pedicles," also developed about the same time by ophthalmologists (eye specialists)

Filatov of Odessa and Granzer of Berlin (Rogers 1988), better protected the blood supply and enabled surgeons to transfer skin in stages from one location to another. Johannes Fredericus Samuel Esser, an ingenious Dutch surgeon, experimented with epithelial inlays to rebuild eyelids and vascular pedicles to transfer hair-bearing skin for eyebrow reconstructions. Varaztad Kazanjian, an American immigrant from Armenia, was a dentist with two years of medical school when he joined the Harvard unit of the British Army Medical Corps. He established the first maxillofacial treatment center in France where he wired fragments of jaws together, developed specialized facial and dental prosthetics, and invented internal rubber splints to prevent faces from contracting until more extensive bone grafting could be done. Other American surgeons also went overseas to help and to learn. Vilray Blair, an experienced surgeon with a long résumé of articles and a book on surgery of the mouth and jaw before the war, was named chief of the Armed Forces' plastic surgery section. He returned from Gillies's facility to organize teams of medical and dental surgeons to care for the wounded (Hait 1994). He directed one of the three U.S. military hospitals eventually designated for plastic surgery patients—Jefferson Barracks in Missouri. His assistant, Robert Ivy, headed the team assigned to Walter Reed Hospital. George Shaeffer headed the unit at Ft. McHenry in Baltimore where John Staige Davis trained many of the surgeons.

Despite the considerable progress in reconstructive techniques, there were limits to what surgeons could do for the most severely maimed. Some devised unique prosthetics for such patients to help restore function and a more normal appearance. In those relatively few patients for whom both surgery and prosthetics proved inadequate, artists fashioned elaborate facial masks to hide the worst of their deformities. But what could be accomplished by a skillful surgeon trained in the emerging techniques of plastic surgery was acclaimed as a modern miracle by the media. By the end of the war, these surgeons had earned the respect of their colleagues and the public. No longer were questions raised about the morality of surgical reconstruction or, for that matter, about the social value of medical practice.

Organization and Professionalization

The respect gained by surgeons during the First World War was part of a larger transformation underway in American medicine. Abraham Flexner's 1910 study of medical schools, sponsored by the Carnegie Foundation, deplored the inadequate training of most practicing physicians, a legacy of the medical "counterculture" of the nineteenth century (Starr 1982). Neither medical education nor medical practice was regulated at that time. Most medical schools were proprietary with no entrance standards, no laboratories, and no clinical training. Anyone could claim to be a physician. While most "regular," allopathic, physicians embraced germ theory and abandoned the most baseless heroic therapies, "irregulars" continued to espouse a variety of alternative theories about the origin and appropriate treatment of disease.

At the time of the war, the small but vocal American Medical Association (AMA) was engaged in a vitriolic campaign against patent-medicine manufacturers, magnetic healers, homeopaths, chiropractors, osteopaths, midwives, "beauty doctors," and other irregulars whom the organization branded as quacks. The AMA also sought to organize regular physicians into a tightly bound profession. It used the Flexner report to argue for control over the admission standards, length, and, most important, scientific rigor of medical education and for state licensure laws to regulate who could practice medicine. The transformation took several decades. As a result, the boundary between quackery and legitimate medicine was blurred in the early decades of the twentieth century, but the era of unregulated, proprietary medical schools and self-proclaimed physicians was waning after World War I.

The respect gained by the reconstructive work of surgeons in World War I supported the AMA's quest for public recognition of the legitimate complexity of medicine and the need to "protect" patients with regulation of medical training and practice under its authority. Tight regulation also would eventually provide the newly consolidating profession some protection from competitors. Maintaining such a powerful occupational privilege depended on the new profession's commitment to the continued development of its specialized body of knowledge about health care, based on medical science, and its use of this knowledge to serve the public good.

Information about innovations in medicine, then as now, spread through medical journals and presentations at meetings sponsored by organizations of physicians with similar interests. These formal organizations institutionalized the division of labor that already existed in the emerging profession. The increasingly rapid expansion of medical knowledge since the latter part of the nineteenth century meant that no physician could be an expert in all areas. Nor was it necessary, because most common health problems could be adequately managed by general practitioners. Some physicians, however, chose to concentrate in areas such as surgery, otolaryngology, ophthalmology, gynecology, and pediatrics. Innovations in knowledge, techniques, and tools created still more areas of specialization and new organizations. Sociologists such as Sydney Halpern (1988, 4–9) argue that these structural segments function as professions within a profession. Specialty organizations added to their mission the codification of the knowledge and experience that practitioners in their areas should have. These guidelines shaped the evolving curricula of medical schools and, eventually, residency programs. These guidelines also provided the criteria used by voluntary programs set up by the specialties to certify physicians who met their criteria.

Certification by a specialty review board has become the norm in the United States, although it remains voluntary and does not impose a legal restriction on the practice of any licensed physician. Specialty certification, however, is often a critical criterion for gaining hospital privileges and for contracting with managed care plans.

Some of the surgeons who gained experience in reconstructive surgery during the First World War felt the need for an organization to nurture their nascent specialty. Three met in Chicago in 1921 and elected twenty surgeons as founding members of the American Association of Oral Surgeons (Goldwyn 1990a). The organization's first name reflects its original focus on the maxillofacial problems of the war years. Membership required both medical and dental degrees, although exceptions were made for Chalmers Lyons, who only had a dental degree, and Vilray Blair, who had only a medical degree, in recognition of their extensive wartime maxillofacial experience. Few others could meet the dual degree requirements of this exclusive association and the dental degree requirement was dropped two years later. This decision located the new specialty firmly within medicine, rather than at the border of medicine and dentistry. The organization's name was broadened to American Association of Oral and Plastic Surgeons in 1937 and finally changed to its present name, the American Association of Plastic Surgeons, in 1942.

The American Association of Plastic Surgeons, like other specialty organizations, began as a forum for the exchange of information between members at meetings and then enlarged its mission to include formal training programs. It launched the American Board of Plastic

Surgery in 1937 to establish standards for certification as a specialist in plastic surgery. The 1941 admission of this board to the AMA's Advisory Board of Medical Specialties (the precursor to the American Board of Medical Specialties) solidified the small new specialty's independent status. Membership in the elite American Association of Plastic Surgeons remains by invitation only. From the beginning, the association was closely linked with the directors of plastic surgery training programs in university-based medical schools and it grew as the number of these programs increased.

The exclusivity of the association led other physicians to consider forming a more open organization for all practitioners of plastic surgery (Hait 1994). One of the instigators was Jacques Maliniac, a Polish Jew who went to medical school at the University of Paris and tended the wounded on the Balkan front during World War I before immigrating to the United States. Although he was instrumental in establishing an independent plastic surgery service at a municipal hospital in New York, he was not asked to join the association, perhaps because of his notoriously difficult personality or perhaps because of his relatively open practice of cosmetic surgery, a practice which was disdained by most members of the association. Nevertheless, he succeeded in establishing the Society of Plastic and Reconstructive Surgery in 1931 to provide an open forum for all practitioners engaged in plastic surgery, information to members of other specialties interested in plastic problems, and public education about the new specialty. The group was small and heterogeneous. Like the original members of the association, the first members of the society had varied backgrounds; four of the first five chairmen of the society after Maliniac were board-certified otolaryngologists and the other was an ophthalmologist. All, however, were committed to the development of a separate new specialty, rather than to the absorption of plastic techniques by their previous specialties.

At first the small society mainly facilitated meetings for east coast practitioners excluded by the American Association of Plastic Surgeons. In spite of the society's original role as an alternative to the academics' association, the two evolved into sibling organizations with different functions; the latter concentrates on training programs and the former represents the other occupational interests of the specialists, including, as will be seen in subsequent chapters, sponsoring meetings, disseminating new information, and lobbying legislators on issues of interest to members. In the early 1940s the society had 101 members, including members of the academic association who eventually took over the leadership of the society. It changed its name to the American Society of Plastic and Reconstructive Surgeons (ASPRS). Membership was restricted to only board-certified plastic surgeons in America and comparably qualified foreign plastic surgeons.

The small but aggressive ASPRS launched a full-scale specialty journal, *Plastic and Reconstructive Surgery,* immediately after World War II. Within a year the periodical had almost twelve hundred domestic and foreign subscriptions. It became the world's premier plastic surgery journal and the official publication of both the association and the ASPRS as well as several subspecialty organizations including the American Society of Maxillofacial Surgeons, a group that specializes in lower face problems. The ASPRS has become the most visible and powerful organization of plastic surgeons in the world. The organization changed its name again in the fall of 1999 to the American Society of Plastic Surgeons.

Modern Innovation

If the seeds of plastic surgery were the ancient Indian and fifteenth- and sixteenth-century Italian use of flaps to rebuild mutilated noses, the roots were composed of the innovative techniques for facial reconstruction demanded by the trench warfare of World War I. Once these roots were firmly established, the new hybrid specialty grew vigorously in several directions. Not only were plastic surgeons regarded as the experts for reconstruction of facial trauma and congenital malformations, but also their refinement of grafting techniques gave them authority over treating burns and difficult wounds anywhere on the body. Blair and Brown's split thickness innovation led Earl Padgett to develop the dermatome with the assistance of George Hood, a mechanical engineer. This tool, introduced in 1939, produced calibrated split-thickness skin grafts. It saved many lives and limbs in World War II because it made it possible to transplant large amounts of skin rapidly (Rogers 1988, 144). The moving ground action of the Second World War, combined with the extensive use of land mines, produced many leg injuries and large gaping wounds that were difficult to heal. Healing such wounds had become a higher priority after blood transfusions and antibiotics greatly increased the chances of survival among the injured. Most plastic surgeons had already adopted John Staige Davis's technique for wound closure using Z incisions, a technique which he presented at the 1938 ASPRS meeting (Hait 1994, 19A). This technique, together with generous amounts of skin grafting, greatly improved outcomes.

Following the Second World War plastic surgeons turned their attention to new challenges. Other physicians referred their most difficult wounds, bed sores, and burns to plastic surgeons. Many used their skills to excise complicated and large tumors and repair the resulting wounds. Some focused on hand surgery using the multi-specialty team model adopted during the war. Others were involved in the early development of organ transplantation. The *Transplantation Bulletin* merged with *Plastic and Reconstructive Surgery* from 1957 to 1961, and plastic surgeon Joseph Murray was awarded a Nobel prize for his work on kidney transplants in the 1970s.

Important advances continued in the treatment of trauma and congenital anomalies (Hait 1994). Ralph Millard and Kerwin Marks developed better approaches to cleft palate and cleft lip repair. Milton Adams devised an internal technique to wire together facial bone fractures in the middle third of the face. Bone grafts were used successfully to reconstruct lower jaws. Some advances were revolutionary. Myocutaneous flaps improved outcomes. Innovations in microvascular surgery in the 1960s led to dramatic successes, beginning with replantation of severed fingers and toes. Parisian Paul Tessier and his associates introduced cranial, facial, and orbital osteotomies, adding to plastic surgery the new subspecialty of craniofacial surgery to complement the lower-face subspecialty of maxillofacial surgery. Other technological innovations included tissue expansion, synthetic skin substitutes, vacuum suction, endotracheal anesthesia, and, more recently, endoscopic surgery. Plastic surgeons are now looking for ways to duplicate the scarless healing that takes place in the womb after fetal surgery. The most publicly visible innovations after the Second World War, however, were in the rapidly growing offshoot of cosmetic surgery.

The History of Cosmetic Surgery

Cosmetic surgery's history is intertwined with that of reconstructive surgery. Most of the basic techniques are the same; the difference is the purpose of the surgery. Cosmetic surgery began in the middle of the nineteenth century, before anesthesia, asepsis, and antibiotics, when a few individuals started to seek practitioners willing to try to surgically improve the appearance of a feature that fell within the normal range of variation. Most surgeons at that time regarded such operations as frivolous, if not immoral, given the danger of infection. Nevertheless, some did them discreetly, yielding to the forces of technological imperialism. Only a few published their techniques, and some of these were dismissed by other physicians as incompetent, unethical quacks.

Nineteenth-Century Emergence

As with reconstructive surgery, most of the early cosmetic procedures were done on noses. People came to Dieffenbach, famous for his skillful reconstructive work, and others to build up their "saddle noses" (Rogers 1976). In some cases the saddle shape of a nose was merely a family trait; in others it was a secondary effect of trauma or disease. No matter what the cause, a few were willing to risk surgery and uncertain results because saddle noses in the nineteenth century were associated with syphilis, a highly stigmatized disease. Practitioners experimented with inserting ivory, bone, cartilage, and paraffin, but their efforts were often defeated by the body's immune system. Others risked infection and uncertain results to have their large, hooked, or drooping noses reduced. All had to accept visible scars as part of the price.

External incisions are still used to narrow flared nostrils and in some other procedures, but most rhinoplasty is now done with internal incisions. The American otolaryngologist John Orlando Roe led the way when he used an intranasal approach in 1887 to "correct" a pug nose, a trait stigmatized by its association with the Irish peasants who flooded into the United States after famine engulfed their homeland. Within four years he had extended this technique to reshape the noses of other stigmatized ethnic groups, particularly Jews. Although Roe pioneered intranasal cosmetic surgery, the history of aesthetic rhinoplasty also owes much to the esteemed Jacques Joseph of Berlin. He originated most of the variations and instruments in use today, and by 1905 he had performed one hundred cosmetic operations on noses. More important, he published descriptions of his procedures and documented the outcomes in photographs.

Joseph did other cosmetic procedures as well. A compendium of his plastic surgery articles written from the late 1890s through the early 1900s included two chapters on surgery of the forehead and eyelids. He later revealed that he had experimented with excisions of excess skin in other areas of the face. He was not the first to report the removal of excess skin folds of the eyelids, but he was, along with Charles C. Miller of Chicago and Frederick Strange Kolle of New York, among the first to focus on aesthetic considerations of this surgery. Other cosmetic procedures reported in the nineteenth century included the reduction of protruding ears, documented by Edward Talbot Ely in 1881, and the use of acids such as phenol to peel the upper layers of skin to reduce wrinkles and blemishes.

Beauty Surgeons in the Early Twentieth Century

After the turn of the century, a few physicians in Europe and the United States began to experiment with numerous small excisions of excess skin to reduce overall facial wrinkles and double chins. The results tended to be mixed and short-term. The injection of pure paraffin and paraffin mixtures to fill facial wrinkles and gaunt cheeks was more common. A few experimented with injecting paraffin and other substances into women's breasts. As with its use to build up saddle noses, the initial good results were followed by serious problems (Goldwyn 1980b). The substances tended to migrate and many patients developed paraffinomas, also known as wax cancers. These cancers were difficult to remove and left patients scarred. Other problems included thrombosis, phlebitis, and pulmonary embolisms. There also were attempts in the 1920s and 1930s to transplant fatty tissue from women's abdomens and buttocks into their breasts, but initial good cosmetic results were followed by a high rate of liquefaction and absorption (Schalk 1988). Others tried inserting ivory and glass balls, although the cosmetic results were far from satisfactory.

Muckraking journalists in the early twentieth century deplored paraffin use and the increasingly common practices of face peeling and cosmetic surgery in beauty parlors, offices, and hotel rooms. At the same time the AMA was in the midst of its campaign to organize regular physicians and eliminate irregular quacks, including beauty doctors, "featural specialists," and others. Despite the resistance of the emerging profession of medicine, cosmetic surgery continued to grow slowly. The culture was changing.

A more secular, consumer culture tied to industrialization, democratization, and modernization eroded the Victorian emphasis on inner qualities of character. "Good looks," rather than "good works," became the consuming concern of adolescent girls (Brumberg 1997). For women, the notion that beauty radiated from internal goodness, spirituality, and self-control mutated into the idea that every woman could look beautiful with a little self-discipline and the help of the new, commercial, beauty industry. A proliferation of beauty advice columns promoted a cultural imperative for women of all ages to pursue self-improvement in appearance. This industry advertised a burgeoning array of cosmetic products, ranging from lotions and makeup to false hair pieces and dyes. Cosmetic surgery, although much less common, was as much a part of this industry as manicures and electrolysis.

In the first few decades of the twentieth century, before organized medicine had succeeded in establishing tight control over the practice of medicine and restrictions on advertising, entrepreneurial practitioners advertised their cosmetic surgery services in urban newspapers, women's magazines, and brochures. A few others relied on public relations efforts, including articles and books, to recruit patients. Charles Miller was an example of the latter (Haiken 1997, 25–29). In addition to numerous articles, he published the first book devoted exclusively to cosmetic surgery in 1907. Not only did he describe procedures to reduce noses and protruding ears and build up depressed noses, he also described operations to lift foreheads and eyelids. Moreover, he discussed how to remove crow's feet, bags under eyes, and double chins, create dimples, change the size of lips, and prevent expression lines by severing specific facial nerves. Although his publications contained many illustrations, he included no photographs to document his outcomes. He was regarded by most regular physicians of his day as a self-aggrandizing quack. In hindsight, it could be argued that he was a surgical visionary. He perceptively recognized that the increasing attention given to physical beauty in twentieth-century newspapers and women's magazines was the driving force behind the expanding demand for cosmetic surgery and, combined with advertising, opened the door to exploitation. He decried the incompetent, "unscrupulous charlatans" who victimized gullible patients and implored ethical surgeons to take patients' cosmetic requests seriously. He also anticipated the mental health rationale that would be adopted later in the century to justify cosmetic surgery's eventual inclusion within regular medicine.

Miller was not alone in justifying cosmetic surgery in terms of a patient's psychological health. Adalbert Bettman, a regular physician in Oregon, for example, enthusiastically promoted the idea that cosmetic surgery improved a person's sense of well-being. Rogers (1976) credits him with the 1919 introduction of the more extensive incisions that became the standard facelift procedure until the late 1970s. While others talked of "imperfections" and "correcting" appearances, Bettman (1988) defined wrinkles and double chins as "deformities." He even suggested that they were more cruel for his women patients than the loss of a leg.

Other respected practitioners, such as Maliniac, defended their cosmetic work in terms of the social impact and economic repercussions of appearance. The widespread belief that restoration of the appearance of soldiers maimed in World War I was a worthy goal paved the way for such a rationale, as did the proliferation of images of attractive, successful people in movies and magazines after the war. Most regular physicians willing to do cosmetic surgery extrapolated a justification for their work from the maxim "One's face is one's fortune."

Most cosmetic surgery in the first few decades of the twentieth century, however, was not done by respected surgeons with training and experience in reconstructive surgery. It was done by beauty doctors, such as Miller, who flourished before organized medicine in the United States succeeded in closing outlets for their advertising and instituting licensure requirements. The beauty doctors also justified their work in terms of the social, economic, and psychological impact of appearance.

Beauty doctors were not solely an American phenomenon. Madame le Dr. A. Noël of France was an early pioneer in facelifting. Working out of her home without a surgical mask or gloves, she also removed bags under eyes, excess skin above eyes, flabby arm tissue, double chins, and reduced protruding ears. Her 1926 book contained pre- and postoperative photographs of her patients, who, Rogers notes, look amazingly good, considering the external incisions. Also in 1926, a Swiss-German, Charles Henry Willi, published a book that he sent to selected "good addresses" in London (Cameron and Wallace 1991). There is no record that he had any formal medical training and only speculation that he may have worked as an orderly for Jacques Joseph in Berlin before coming to London. Nevertheless, he did more than fifteen hundred cosmetic operations by 1949, working out of his home, usually with only local anesthetic. A nurse who worked for him described his results as excellent, but she quit after six months because she worried about the risks of monitoring patients with "no medical cover," not even a means to measure their blood pressure.

Elizabeth Haiken's comparison of the backgrounds and careers of six American surgeons demonstrates the blurred continuum between

quacks and regular physicians in the first four decades of the twentieth century (1997, 55–90). Where practitioners were located on this
continuum had less to do with the rigor of their training and skill than
with their reputation in the eyes of those committed to organized medicine. At one extreme were men such as Vilray Blair and Jacques
Maliniac, whose extensive reconstructive work in World War I earned
professional respect and the right to shape the newly organizing specialty. Cosmetic surgery was only a small portion of their practices
and not an area of work they actively sought or publicized. They were
opposed to public self-promotion, although the press occasionally
quoted them as experts. But it is worth repeating that even Maliniac,
founder of the ASPRS, encountered resistance from his plastic surgeon
colleagues, probably in part because he was more open about his
cosmetic work than most regular practitioners.

In the middle of the spectrum were men such as Joseph Eastman
Sheehan and Maxwell Maltz, whose training at elite schools and recognized skills were overshadowed by image problems. Sheehan, a
member of the AMA and the American Association of Plastic Surgeons,
survived a publicized malpractice suit over a facelift in 1927, but was
nearly expelled from the specialty when a 1935 profile in *Time* depicted him as a wealthy dandy who charged exorbitant fees. That controversy, together with a few other dubious alliances, almost derailed
his bid for board certification in plastic surgery. His leadership role
in medical education and continuing commitment to reconstructive
surgery may have saved him.

Maltz, in contrast, was denied certification, even though he was
a member of the AMA, published articles on reconstructive techniques
in respected medical journals, and never generated negative publicity. His attempt to sponsor a rival society for plastic surgeons in 1934
may have contributed to his rejection. His office in an area of New
York City that *Vogue* called the essential neighborhood for women interested in beauty surely tainted him, as did his association with show
business personalities. Although he did not advertise, he sought personal publicity in other ways. He volunteered his reconstructive services to the poor and to young criminals who were disfigured, believing
that he could rebuild their character by rebuilding their faces. Articles
about his work appeared in *Cosmopolitan* and *Esquire.* He published
four autobiographical books, a novel about a plastic surgeon, a play
that a critic described as a vanity production, and a fictionalized
biography of Tagliacozzi. Such blatant self-promotion was discouraged

by organized medicine, but it proved to be an effective way to recruit patients. Toward the end of his surgical career, Maltz changed his focus to publishing self-help books and achieved considerable fame and fortune with his psycho-cybernetics program that combined self-image psychology and self-hypnosis. In the final analysis, Maltz was more commercial in his orientation and more connected to cosmetic work than Sheehan. He was blackballed by colleagues anxious to establish an unimpeachable image for the small new specialty.

At the other extreme of the spectrum were the beauty doctors who aggressively solicited patients. Few had much formal training. Most practiced outside the emerging boundaries of organized, professional medicine. Henry Junius Schireson and J. Howard Crum belonged to this group. Plastic surgeons today, if they have heard of the two men, feel no kinship with them. They did not join medical societies. They did not have hospital privileges. They did not publish in medical journals. They did not teach at medical schools. Yet, Haiken persuasively argues that these flamboyant irregular practitioners shaped the early public perception of plastic surgery more than did regular practitioners because they dominated news coverage of plastic surgery.

Schireson attained national renown in 1923 when he operated on vaudeville star Fanny Brice's nose. The intense press coverage made the American people, even those living in small towns and rural areas, aware of this type of cosmetic surgery. In 1927 he was back in the news with other procedures. He sued a British actress and her mother for allegedly failing to pay for facelifts and claimed to have reshaped American showgirl Peaches Browning's legs. Fame turned into infamy the next year in Illinois when his attempt to straighten a young woman's bow legs resulted in gangrene and a double amputation. He lost his Illinois license, but resurfaced in the news a decade later in a posh Philadelphia area when he published a book on plastic surgery. Shortly thereafter he was indicted and convicted for fraud and perjury in a bankruptcy declaration filed in the face of mounting malpractice lawsuits and debts. Subsequent investigation by newspaper reporters uncovered previous convictions for selling narcotics in Baltimore, conspiracy to defraud, and practicing medicine without a license in New York. Once again Schireson resumed practice after his release from prison in 1942 and delayed efforts by Pennsylvania to revoke his license for five more years. The man the AMA and *Time* called the "King of Quacks" died less than two years later, after a forty-year career as a beauty doctor.

Like Schireson, Crum viewed publicity as the door to a successful

practice. He published two books. He actively cultivated press attention and advertised in newspapers and telephone directories. He also
lectured on cosmetic surgery at New York department stores. His most
successful publicity efforts were far more theatrical and, consequently,
deemed newsworthy by the press. In front of an audience estimated
to be between six hundred and fifteen hundred in a hotel ballroom,
Crum lifted the face of a sixty-year-old character actress under a local
anesthetic at the 1931 International Beauty Shop Owners Convention.
The intrepid woman had her hair waved and her photograph taken
after bandages were applied. At the same convention the next year,
more than one thousand women watched Crum do a "type-changing"
operation. Echoing contemporary ideas in criminology and physiognomy, Crum claimed he would transform a released convict into a
law-abiding citizen by changing her face. Five years later he operated
on the flat noses of three Honduran family members in a vaudeville-
type of performance. It was probably Crum who operated in front of
one thousand beauty experts in New York about two years later. This
time the patient selected a face to suit her personality and a pianist
played beauty-themed music during the operation.

The antics of the publicity-driven, reckless, and unethical
Schireson and the showman Crum helped regular physicians—general
practitioners and specialists alike—define norms for their consolidating profession. Those specializing in plastic surgery knew that the fate
of their fledgling field in the United States depended on distancing
plastic surgery from the garish, exploitative, commercial beauty industry and embedding it in the emerging, noncommercial, service-oriented
profession of medicine. Reconstructive applications of plastic surgery
presented no problem; cosmetic applications created a serious dilemma.
While the number of cosmetic operations undoubtedly continued to increase, the trained plastic surgeons who replaced the turn-of-the-century
beauty doctors put cosmetic surgery in medicine's "closet."

Changing Public Views between
the World Wars

The discussion of cosmetic surgery in women's
magazines provides a historical record of changing views, although it
is neither factually accurate, fully consistent, nor frequent. After the
extensive press coverage of Fanny Brice's nose job and news reports
of facelifts, columnist Celia Cole warned *Delineator* readers in 1926

that such operations often turned out poorly and were too dangerous and impermanent to risk for vanity. She advised them not to consider cosmetic surgery, unless they were obsessed with a "really hideous feature." Although her intent was to deter women from cosmetic surgery, she expressed fewer qualms about acid skin peels and the use of ultraviolet rays by a specialist, such as the dermatologist she interviewed for the article.

The next year Joseph Bloodgood, a professor of medicine at the citadel of regular medicine—Johns Hopkins—offered *Delineator* readers a more positive perspective of cosmetic surgery (1927). Although he cautioned readers about its dangers, he affirmed its potential to improve appearance. His claim that the dangers had less to do with the type of operation than with the qualifications and ethics of the surgeon foreshadowed the specialty's central theme in the latter part of the century. He warned readers to avoid the many unscrupulous beauty surgeons who would operate on anyone who could pay. He advised them to go to a plastic surgeon who would judge whether surgery was appropriate.

The idea that a surgeon would turn away prospective paying patients whose appearance flaws were not severe enough, or could not be improved sufficiently, to warrant the risks of surgery lies at the heart of Bloodgood's conception of an ethical practice and the difference between a commercial and a professional service. He expressed no prejudice against cosmetic applications of plastic surgery to the readers unlike most regular physicians in the emergent profession. Journalist Richard Walsh that same year similarly reassured *Woman's Home Companion* readers that they had a right to look good and advised that there were a few ethical surgeons offering cosmetic surgery along with many unethical and incompetent surgeons (1927). Echoing the AMA campaign against quacks, he warned that the stringency of state medical licensure laws differed widely and that advertising claims by practitioners were unregulated and unreliable.

Writer Dorothy Cocks elaborated on the ethical problems of advertising and, more generally, promoting medical services as a commercial product in a 1930 *Good Housekeeping* article. She told readers that advertising was the sign of a flagrant charlatan and that self-promotion in public presentations, newspaper and magazine articles, and books was the mark of a semi-charlatan. She did not condemn cosmetic surgery; she only condemned the commercialization of it and advised interested readers to seek one of the few plastic surgeons with wartime reconstructive experience who eschewed both advertising and public self-promotion. Only they could be trusted.

At the same time that Cocks condemned advertising in *Good Housekeeping, Vogue* continued to publish advertisements for beauty doctors along with other commercial beauty services and products at the back of the magazine. Here readers could find practitioners offering facelifts, wrinkle removal, and surgical modifications of the nose, ears, and breasts. *Vogue* explicitly assured readers that the advertisers could be trusted. These advertisements continued throughout the 1930s. By 1939, however, the AMA's campaign to stop individual physician advertising and self-promotion had gained ground. A *Ladies Home Journal* editor informed readers of Gretta Palmer's "When Plastic Surgery Is Justified" that no surgeons' names were included because the "profession" opposed anything verging on advertising (1939). Classified advertisements for surgery disappeared from *Vogue* about this time.

At the end of the 1930s, the message about cosmetic surgery in women's magazines, as in other magazines and newspapers, was both more complex and more tolerant. Articles like one in a 1939 *Ladies Home Journal* alerted readers to new cosmetic operations to widen eyes and change the size and shape of lips. Most also warned about risks and incompetent practitioners. But the question of why a healthy person would risk surgery to enhance a normal appearance gradually was replaced with the question, "Why not?" Authors, such as Ruth Murrin in a 1940 *Good Housekeeping* article on nose operations, were more likely to tell readers that an unattractive appearance was a handicap and that cosmetic surgery could transform a person's life than to suggest that it built character. Even minor flaws could undermine self-esteem and no longer need be tolerated, according to Lois Miller's 1939 *Independent Woman* article.

The Schism in Plastic Surgery

Haiken suggests that plastic surgeons had to absorb cosmetic surgery—procedures and ideology—to assert control over their specialty because of public demand for it. While the specialty rooted in reconstructive surgery did eventually acknowledge cosmetic surgery as legitimate work for its members, it did so only with great reluctance, internal dissension, a little hypocrisy, and considerable rationalization. The outcome could have been different. Medicine's mandate is to heal, not to beautify. Public demand for beautification was not sufficient to medicalize appearance. At least some regular physicians had to be willing to accommodate the demand. The transformation of American medicine from an unregulated free market at the beginning of the twentieth century into an organized, self-regulated institution with rigorous control over the admission criteria and content of medical education and professional licensure drove most irregular practitioners out of business, including the likes of Schireson and Crum. Eventually all states required graduation from an accredited medical school and successful performance on a licensure examination to practice medicine. Because organized medicine won control of the accreditation of medical schools, the content of licensure examinations, and the definition of what constitutes the practice of medicine, there could be no cosmetic surgery unless some regular physicians in organized medicine were willing to offer it.

At least a few regular physicians had been willing to do cosmetic surgery since the middle of the nineteenth century, even if they were reluctant to discuss it. European-born practitioners in New York like Maliniac and Gustave Aufricht, both of whom trained with Joseph in Berlin, were generally more forthcoming about their cosmetic work. Nevertheless, they fought to separate themselves from the beauty doctors. Gustav Tieck, another New York practitioner, waited until 1920 to report that he had done more than one thousand rhinoplasties because he wanted to make sure that he had "placed this branch of surgery on a definite scientific basis" (cited in Haiken 1997, 35, 39). Like most other regular physicians willing to do cosmetic surgery at that time, he said he was only willing to operate on patients whose appearance was deviant enough to cause "'serious social or business embarrassment."

After the war other regular physicians, including the highly respected Blair and Kazanjian, quietly applied their reconstructive skills to some cosmetic cases, but they publicly continued to express concern about the place of cosmetic surgery in professional medicine. Blair (1936) resented patients asking plastic surgeons to operate on minor defects. He believed that catering to frivolous vanities belittled the profession and violated orthodox medical ethics. The highly influential John Staige Davis, author of the first comprehensive text on plastic surgery in 1919, was more adamant in his opposition. He stated that Johns Hopkins surgeons were not interested in either the development or performance of cosmetic surgery. He articulated the sentiments of many others when he asserted, "True plastic surgery . . . is absolutely distinct and separate from what is known as cosmetic or decorative surgery" (Davis 1926, 203). The latter is "unessential," while the former is "'necessary to the health of the patient." This distinction lies at the heart of the current definition adopted by the specialty and by the AMA.

Acutely aware of the importance of image for the new specialty's quest for respect and a legitimate place in the emerging profession of medicine in the early twentieth century, plastic surgeons who did cosmetic surgery did it on the side, out of view. This practice continued in large part until the 1970s, despite an increasing volume of rhinoplasties and face- and eye lifts. Some operated out of hospital; others operated under false diagnoses (Rees 1991). They worked surreptitiously because they knew that many of their professional colleagues, especially those who were not plastic surgeons, still considered cosmetic work an ethically questionable use of medical skills.

The academic leadership of the ASPRS was committed to downplaying cosmetic surgery. Only rarely did a paper presented at the annual meetings address a cosmetic procedure. Those that did were usually on nose surgery, which, for patients with extremely unattractive noses, was more acceptable in the eyes of many physicians than facial rejuvenation (Hait 1994). Plastic surgeons who submitted papers on cosmetic subjects were repeatedly rejected (Webster 1984, 8). The same was true for papers submitted to *Plastic and Reconstructive Surgery*. Similarly, when medical schools added plastic surgery residencies in the 1950s, few procedures other than reconstructive were covered.

"Outing" Cosmetic Surgery

In spite of the institutionalized schism between reconstructive and cosmetic surgery, by the 1960s cosmetic surgery had become the cornerstone of many established plastic surgeons' private practices and a lucrative sideline for those on medical school faculties. The combination of techniques these experienced plastic surgeons used were still shrouded in secrecy. Younger plastic surgeons charged that established practitioners would not share their expertise because they wanted to protect their personal financial interests. The esteemed professional image and legitimacy of medicine were taken for granted by young plastic surgeons in the 1960s, unlike their older colleagues who remembered the early decades of the twentieth century. The authority and legitimacy of the modern medical profession was firmly established, and plastic surgery had been an officially recognized specialty within this profession since 1941. In contrast, appearance was more important than ever before and the demand for cosmetic surgery was accelerating, even though it was not highly visible.

Two of the younger plastic surgeons, Thomas Baker and Howard Gordon, organized a Symposium on Cosmetic Surgery in 1961 (*Plastic Surgery News* 1994b). They argued that, unless plastic surgeons taught cosmetic surgery, it could "drift into the back water of commercialism and be dispensed indiscriminately" (Murray and Baker 1970, 389). The Miami symposium, which included live demonstrations, was immensely successful and became an annual event. Some American plastic surgeons also attended seminars on cosmetic surgery organized by Mario Gonzalez-Ulloa in Mexico City in the 1960s and 1970s, over the objections of the ASPRS leadership (Webster 1984, 8). However, these opportunities were not enough to satiate physician interest in cosmetic techniques, innovations, and outcomes.

Some disgruntled plastic surgeons, led by Simon Fredricks and John Lewis, formed the American Society for Aesthetic Plastic Surgery in 1967. Like the ASPRS, this society requires board certification in plastic surgery. Hait (1994) reports that ASPRS leadership feared that this new organization would splinter the ASPRS membership. If it had, the power of plastic surgeons, already one of the smallest specialties, would have been diminished greatly. The ASPRS avoided this fate by officially recognizing the aesthetic society as a sister organization in 1969, despite the concerns and objections of some "old guard" members. To solidify its status as a sister organization, the aesthetic society also requires membership in the ASPRS. By 1999 the society had 1,384 members.

The ASPRS succeeded in preserving its umbrella of structural unity over plastic surgeons, but the organization was transformed. The aesthetic society wielded enough power to break the control of academic plastic surgeons and elect one of its own as secretary of the ASPRS in 1969. The next year the group succeeded in electing a high-profile cosmetic surgeon to the vice presidency, and he subsequently assumed the presidency. Elections became political contests rather than tributes to members of the elite inner circle of academics. The inner circle was invaded and the invaders were determined to bring cosmetic surgery "out of the closet." Once out, physicians were more willing to discuss their work with journalists who were eager to cover the topic. Patient demand boomed.

The aesthetic society not only gave plastic surgeons a special forum to exchange information about cosmetic developments, but also, with help from members elected to leadership positions in the ASPRS, forced open the ASPRS meetings and journal to more papers on cosmetic procedures. The stigma of cosmetic surgery eroded considerably. Cosmetic textbooks followed in the 1970s. The society also produced videotapes and workshops on specific procedures. Young plastic surgeons finally had access to the information they wanted.

Otolaryngologists interested in cosmetic procedures encountered similar opposition from the leaders of their specialty. A few sought training elsewhere and established courses for others. Several small societies of practitioners who did cosmetic surgery were formed. Faced with strong opposition from the well-organized ASPRS, discussed in the next chapter, these groups eventually merged into the American Academy of Facial Plastic and Reconstructive Surgery in 1964 (Simons and Hill 1989). Training was largely informal. Otolaryngologists' interest in cosmetic surgery grew as antibiotics and other drugs reduced the infections that had been a large part of their work. The future of otolaryngology as a unified specialty was in doubt. The field was breaking into many subspecialties ranging from bronchology to otology, each with its own academic society. By the mid-1960s there were more than a dozen subspecialty groups. In the middle of this fragmentation, the American Academy of Facial Plastic and Reconstructive Surgery won approval for its first aging face course in 1969. Then the academy lobbied, over the opposition of the plastic surgeons, to include soft tissue training in residencies. By 1975 facial plastic surgery training was a mandatory part of an otolaryngology residency. Plastic surgeons were unable to stop the academy from securing a seat in the AMA's powerful House of Delegates in 1978 and from convincing the AMA to include "'facial plastic surgery" on its physician self-designated specialty list in 1985. The American Academy of Facial Plastic and Reconstructive Surgery published its first book on cosmetic surgery of the face in 1984 and its first consumer book, *The Face Book*, in 1988. In 1999 under the auspices of the AMA the academy launched its own specialty journal, *Archives of Facial Plastic Surgery.* Plastic surgeons immediately complained they were not consulted and tried unsuccessfully to stipulate that the journal be discontinued if unprofitable within two years.

Innovations

Some significant technical developments in cosmetic surgery took place in the 1950s and 1960s (Webster 1984). Aufricht and Millard contributed new ways of thinking about facelifts. Others experimented with chin implants, dermabrasion, chemical peels, and hair transplants. Several kinds of synthetic sponge breast implants were developed, tried, and abandoned when long term results were unnatural and complications such as fluid accumulation were frequent (Schalk 1988). Outside the United States, plastic surgeons introduced new procedures for thigh lifting, abdominoplasty, and other kinds of body-contouring surgery.

Not all innovations proved safe. Some physicians, including nonplastic surgeons, in the United States, Mexico, and Japan injected liquid silicone to plump up facial wrinkles, acne scars, and breasts (Hait 1994). As with paraffin at the turn of the century, initial good results were followed by serious complications when the silicone migrated. Plastic surgeons were confronted with disfigured patients in the mid-1960s and early 1970s. They initiated a study of liquid silicone outcomes, requested that the Food and Drug Administration (FDA) investigate, and lobbied for state legislatures to outlaw the practice. Their actions pressured the Dow Corning Corporation to withdraw its request for FDA approval of liquid silicone. Doctors turned to collagen and fat injections to plump up wrinkles, scars, and, in the 1990s, lips and the backs of hands. The results, however, only last a few months to a year in most patients due to absorption and must be repeated periodically to maintain the effect.

Other procedures to reduce wrinkles, acne scars, and pigment variations include chemical peels, dermabrasion, dermaplaning, and laser resurfacing. Unlike injectables, which plump up the skin's surface, these procedures remove it. The new skin surface formed in the healing process is smoother, tighter, and younger looking. Phenol is still used for deep layer peels. Its chemical burn reduces coarse wrinkles and scars and the results last longer, although recovery can take from several weeks to several months. Trichloroacetic acid peels have a shorter recovery period but are effective only on more shallow wrinkles. The newest innovation, alpha hydroxy acids, produces only a light peel, but over time it is sufficient to reduce superficial wrinkles and pigmentary changes. Dermabrasion and dermaplaning use tools, rather than chemicals, to remove surface skin. The former involves scraping away the outer layer with a rough wire brush or rotating burr, while the latter uses a dermatome, the device invented to harvest skin for grafting, to shave away the upper layers. Laser resurfacing, the most recent innovation, produces less bleeding, bruising, and postoperative discomfort than the stronger chemical peels, dermabrasion, and dermaplaning, although burns can result. Long-term effects are unknown at this time.

Breast augmentation was revolutionized by the introduction of enclosed silicone breast implants in 1963. The first of these was developed by Dow Corning in cooperation with plastic surgeons Thomas Cronin and Frank Gerow (Schalk 1988). The original design and insertion technique were modified in numerous ways over the next three decades to try to reduce hardening from scar formation, known as capsular contraction. In spite of this frequent undesirable outcome and a high rate of infection, hematoma, displacement, leakage, and rupture, women flocked to physicians for augmentation in the 1970s and 1980s. At the time of the 1990 congressional hearing on the dangers of silicone breast implants, two years before the FDA announced a moratorium on their cosmetic use, an estimated two million women had implants in the United States (U.S. House 1990, 1). Saline implants, fat transfer, and other alternatives, such as peanut oil implants, have taken their place, while surgeons and other researchers conduct required outcomes studies.

Solid silicone has been used to produce an ever expanding array of implants that are useful in both reconstructive and cosmetic applications. These implants have not been associated with the problems of liquid or gel silicone, although they carry the usual surgical risks of anesthetic reaction, infection, scar formation, and bleeding and can move out of place. Cosmetic applications include augmentation of depressed noses, cheek bones, chins, and jaws. They can be contoured to an individual's specific desires and can produce dramatic changes in facial appearance.

Radically different facelifting procedures were introduced in the late 1970s. Instead of merely tightening lax skin that would soon stretch again, surgeons began to separate the skin and tighten the underlying face and neck muscles by repositioning and reducing them. They also reduce or redistribute accumulated fat before redraping and trimming the skin. This "SMAS" procedure has a higher risk of facial nerve damage than mere skin lifts, but it produces a taut, youthful jaw line that, according to ASPRS literature, lasts five to ten years and minimizes scar formation by placing less tension on skin incisions. Sometimes solid silicone implants are added during a facelift to build up the underlying bone structure, and physicians often follow with chemical or laser peels to reduce fine lines. Similarly, other facial rejuvenation procedures—forehead lifts and eyelid surgery—may be done at the same time as a facelift. These have been refined to produce a less hollow look, a well-defined upper eyelid crease, and less visible scars, while correcting frown lines on the forehead, drooping brows and eyelids, and bags under the eyes.

Some surgeons have begun to experiment with endoscopic forehead lifts and, much less frequently, facelifts. The latter are only appropriate for patients without a significant amount of excess skin. Only a small number of short scalp incisions are needed for endoscopy, rather than the standard ear to ear cut across the top of the head in forehead lifts and temple to lower hairline cuts in facelifts. A pencil-sized endoscopic camera inserted through one of the incisions allows the surgeon to view the area beneath the skin on a television monitor. Surgical instruments are inserted through the other incisions to separate the skin and remove or reduce the underlying muscles and tissues to produce a smooth surface. Another new development in the 1990s is the use of botulinum toxin to paralyze the facial muscles that cause deep furrows between the eyes. The idea harks back to Charles Miller, the turn of the century beauty surgeon, who suggested severing some facial muscles.

The introduction of liposuction provided individuals bothered by localized fat deposits an alternative to more extensive body-contouring surgeries such as abdominoplasty and thigh lifts. The original procedure was first described by Joseph Schruddle of Germany in 1972, adapted by Yves-Gérard Illouz of Paris and Giorgio Fischer of Rome in the late 1970s, and imported to the United States in 1982 (Hait 1994). It involves making small incisions in areas with localized fat—abdomen, hips, thighs, buttocks, and "love handles." The surgeon repeatedly thrusts a cannula attached to a pump through these incisions to suction fat in the area.

Plastic surgeons and other physicians involved with cosmetic procedures, ranging from dermatologists to otolaryngologists, packed weekend symposiums to learn about liposuction. A 1983 news article in the *Journal of the American Medical Association* noted that the first ASPRS training course in January of that year attracted three hundred surgeons (Fuerst 1983). Subsequent two- and three-day continuing medical education courses around the country attracted hundreds more. By midyear, the ASPRS resorted to a video symposium of four operations rather than offering a live presentation. The planned enrollment of two hundred had to be doubled to met the intense demand. Despite the lack of hands-on training, the risks of nerve damage, organ perforation, vascular necrosis, shock from heavy fluid loss, infection, and no long-term, follow-up studies, those in attendance expressed a readiness to offer the procedure. Other specialty organizations offered similar workshops and symposiums. No cosmetic practitioner wanted to be left behind. Patients were equally captivated; liposuction became the most frequent cosmetic procedure in the United States before the end of the decade, even though it left many patients with rippled and sometimes discolored skin.

Liposuction, also called lipoplasty by plastic surgeons, has since been modified in a number of ways. Liposculpturing uses smaller cannulas and syringes to suction minor amounts of fat from chins, cheeks, upper arms, abdominal muscles, knees, calves, and ankles. In contrast, the tumescent technique injects liquid containing anesthetic and blood vessel–constricting drugs into the area before suctioning larger fat deposits. The liquid expands the fat compartments and facilitates movement of the cannula beneath the skin. More fat can be suctioned and blood loss and postoperative bruising, swelling, and pain are reduced, compared to standard liposuction. The tumescent procedure's increased risks of pulmonary edema and anesthetic toxicity, however, led some surgeons to develop a more moderate "super-wet" technique in which less liquid and anesthetic is injected. Ultrasound-assisted liposuction also begins with the injection of anesthetic liquid. Then a cannula attached to an ultrasound generator is used to "liquefy" unwanted fat by breaking down the cell walls. The resulting emulsion of fat and liquid is suctioned out of the area. This technique is currently used to remove fat from fibrous body areas such as the back or male breasts, often in conjunction with standard liposuction. Besides the usual risks with liposuction, the skin and deeper tissues can be burned, and fluid collection is more common. The long-term effects of ultrasound-assisted liposuction, like tumescent and standard liposuction, are not yet known. A 1998b ASPRS press release on liposuction mentions five fatalities in the previous few months. Complete national data are not available, although a 1989 congressional hearing on cosmetic surgery referred to eleven deaths in the first seven years of the procedure (U.S.

House 1989a, 1).

There have been numerous other less common cosmetic innovations, some of which remain controversial. For example, starting in the 1980s, pectoral and calf implants, originally developed for reconstruction of disease and trauma-induced deformities, found a new market among bodybuilders and others seeking an athletic physique (Couzens 1992). Many plastic surgeons oppose calf implants as too risky, given the well-known problems of lower leg operations and healing, yet some are willing to do them and to insert prostheses into men's and women's buttocks (González-Ulloa 1991). Even more controversial are penile enlargement operations. Urologists and plastic surgeons sever the suspensory ligament to lengthen the appearance of the penis and inject fat liposuctioned from the abdomen or dermal grafts from the buttocks to thicken it (Taylor 1995). One urologist who advertised penile enlargement aggressively in several state newspapers, in national men's magazines, and on cable television channels reported in court documents that he earned a gross income of $6.6 million in the first six months of 1994. At that point he faced a number of malpractice lawsuits. The most controversial cosmetic developments, however, are controversial not because of health risks, but because of other ethical issues. These include the phenomena of patients with insatiable demands for cosmetic surgery and the surgical modification of racial or ethnic characteristics and the appearance of children with Down's syndrome.

Technological Imperialism, Ethical Dilemma, and the Medicalization of Appearance

Plastic surgery in the Western world has come a long way since the medieval church condemned reconstructive work for interfering with the will of God. And it has come a long way since practitioners felt the need to be circumspect about cosmetic work in order to gain recognition and acceptance of their specialty within the emerging profession of organized medicine. Finally, it has come a long way since practitioners engaged in cosmetic work catered primarily to professional beauties and upper-class women. For reasons discussed in the previous chapter and in chapter 6, cosmetic surgery has democratized. Before that could happen, plastic surgeons had to overcome some ethical dilemmas arising from cosmetic surgery.

Cosmetic surgery poses an ethical dilemma because the cultural authority and professional status granted organized medicine in the early twentieth century is predicated on the occupation's commitment to prevention, diagnosis, and the treatment of disease, trauma, and disability, based on scientific research. Reduced mortality from surgery and infectious diseases paved the way for an expansion of medicine's mandate beyond physiological pathology. Deviant behaviors, such as alcoholism, that eluded control by family, religious, and legal authorities have been medicalized (Conrad and Schneider 1980), as have natural processes that are potentially pathological, such as childbirth (Sullivan and Weitz 1988; Wertz and Wertz 1977) and menopause (Bell 1987; McCrea 1983; Reissman 1983). Cosmetic surgery, like giving synthetic human growth hormone to short children and using steroids to promote muscle development, medicalizes appearance that falls within the normal range of variation. Unlike the medicalization of deviant behaviors and potentially pathological physiological processes, no organic theories are offered to justify the medicalization of appearance. Instead, as Haiken (1997) documents, plastic surgeons embraced cultural ideas about physiognomy and phrenology and the new sciences of psychology and psychiatry. Cosmetic surgery is justified as a medical practice, in the words of an early twentieth-century plastic surgeon, because it can "alleviate or remedy illnesses which in many cases are far more serious than bodily pain; namely mental anguish due to the patient's constant realization of the defect which in turn causes the development of an inferiority complex. . . . Many dependent persons are made self-respecting and self-supporting members of society by the removal of physical and resulting mental handicaps" (Straatsma 1932). Pushed by the forces of technological imperialism and the growing emphasis on appearance, the conceptualization of deformity enlarged to include not only congenital anomalies and the residual effects of disease and trauma, but also the impact of aging and socially undesirable facial features and body contours. Correction of the latter three is justified as "scalpel psychiatry."

The notion of cosmetic surgery as mental health therapy assumes that the cause of the patient's psychological problem is a specific body part, the "correction" of which will improve the patient's self-esteem. The reality is that just over one in five cosmetic patients treated by plastic surgeons are repeat patients and 37 percent have multiple procedures at the same time (American Society of Plastic and Reconstructive Surgeons 1997). The corresponding statistics for members of the American Academy of Cosmetic Surgery (1999) are 27 percent and 32 percent, respectively.

Repeat cosmetic surgery is common because the cosmetic effects of many of the procedures, such as facelifts, have a limited duration. Cosmetic surgery does not stop the impact of aging, lifestyle, or environment. Repeat "rejuvenation" procedures are justified by practitioners as the surgical management of aging, which they view as a disease process. Similarly, multiple procedures are common because surgeons count each procedure separately. A facial rejuvenation that combines a facelift and a forehead lift would be counted as two procedures. There is, however, a gray area between the average cosmetic patient and a group of patients who request modification of one body part after another. These "scalpel slaves" raise concerns among plastic surgeons and other physicians about their appropriate psychological diagnosis and ethical medical treatment. Surgeons who continue to operate on them refer to the ethical principle of autonomy; the principle holds that competent individuals have the right to make decisions about their bodies.

Other questions about Western cultural imperialism, internalized oppression, and, in extreme cases, self-hate are raised about patients who seek to remove obvious indicators of ethnic and racial background (e.g., Gorney 1988; Haiken 1997; Kaw 1993; Rees 1986). Jews began the trend with nose operations before the end of the nineteenth century in reaction to strong anti-Semitic sentiment in Europe and North America (Gilman 1999). Other white minorities with stereotyped noses followed their lead. More recently, nonwhite minorities expanded the scope of surgical change. Asian Americans, who make up an average of 3 percent of plastic surgeons' cosmetic patients (American Society of Plastic and Reconstructive Surgeons 1997), restructure eyelids and noses and enlarge breasts. African Americans, who make up an average of 3 percent of plastic surgeons' cosmetic patients, restructure lips and noses. Michael Jackson, one of the most famous African Americans in the late twentieth century, added other procedures to sculpt a prominent cleft chin and cheekbones. He also may have lightened his skin, although he claims that his dramatic color change is the result of a skin condition. His radical physical transformation prompted considerable public comment both about his motivation and about its unflattering implications regarding the treatment of minorities in American society, as discussed by Haiken (1997).

Anthropologist Eugenia Kaw (1993) argues that the body is central to the experience of racial identity and that members of minority groups internalize a body image reflective of the dominant culture's racial ideology. As a result, they "loathe" those parts of their bodies that caricature their marginal social status, despite claims of racial and ethnic pride. Kaw finds that the explicit motivation for cosmetic surgery among Asian American women is almost always to improve social status rather than mental health. Most surgeons who operate on minority-group patients may be unaware that they are perpetuating inequality and oppression. Instead, they justify these operations in terms of "'objective" aesthetic criteria and the mental health of their patients whose appearance fails to meet these criteria.

The high proportion of women among cosmetic surgery patients raises similar questions about sexism and internalized oppression. Like the "Anglo-Saxonization" of minorities, the surgical "beautification" of women conceptualizes the social problem of discrimination based on appearance as an individual problem of inadequacy and allows the perpetuation of inequality and oppression. Feminists might be expected to politicize the body custom of cosmetic surgery. Susan Bordo (1997) and others do. Most "new feminists," however, do not because they are ideologically reluctant to cast women in the role of passive victims. Instead, they argue that women who seek cosmetic surgery act as "agents" trying to negotiate their bodies and their lives within the constraints of a gendered social order (e.g., Davis 1995). They argue that a woman's decision to have cosmetic surgery is a legitimate solution to the emotional pain she suffers from failing to meet social appearance criteria. Sociologists Diana Dull and Candace West (1991) report that both surgeons and patients also accept the cultural constraints on women and rationalize the decision to have cosmetic surgery as "normal"' and "natural" for women. Concern with appearance is considered essential to women's nature in modern societies. As a result, only rarely is the prevalence of cosmetic surgery among women viewed as problematic. Bordo, in contrast, warns against applying the rhetoric of empowerment to cosmetic surgery because it masks the underlying consumer economy that depends on maintaining a sense of deficiency and need for commercial goods and services. The control that women undergoing cosmetic surgery perceive is an illusion that serves to "up the ante" on acceptable appearance.

One of the most controversial cosmetic surgical practices is the modification of the facial features of children with Down's syndrome. The operation, first reported in Argentina in 1969 and then in the Federal Republic of Germany in 1977, has generated considerable debate

(Dodd and Leahy 1989; Mearig 1989; Sherman 1989; Strauss et al. 1989). Supporters argue that the surgery can reduce the stigma of Down's syndrome by improving function and appearance. Skeptics question whose interests—parent's or child's—are being served, whether psychosocial and behavior modification techniques might be more appropriate, and "who should bear the burden of change, the stigmatized individual or the stigmatizing society" (Katz and Kravetz 1989, 109). They also challenge the effectiveness of the surgery. Initial reports claimed improvements in speech, eating, and appearance, but subsequent research documents complications and fails to find significant improvement in function or appearance when more objective measures than the impressions of involved surgeons and parents are used (Pueschel 1988; Katz and Kravetz 1989). A 1986 British study reports that unrelated nonprofessionals actually rated the children's postoperative appearance as less attractive (Arndt et al., "Fact" 1986). Nevertheless, a survey of board-certified plastic surgeons in Los Angeles and New York City finds that 24 percent have operated on children with Down's and all claim their work was successful; of those who have not, 80 percent would do it to "normalize the appearance to reduce the stigma of mental retardation" (May and Turnbull 1992, 30). In view of the unsupportive outcome data, the continuing cosmetic surgery on children with Down's syndrome is another example of technological imperialism in a society obsessed with appearance.

4 | Medical Entrepreneurs

Market Forces, Regulatory Changes, and the Growth of Cosmetic Surgery

The history of cosmetic surgery shows that technological imperialism within medicine and social and cultural forces outside of medicine have played major roles in the emergence of cosmetic surgery. Yet the high value placed on a pleasing physical appearance is not sufficient to medicalize appearance. For that to happen, at least some physicians must regard appearance as a potential medical problem, conceptualize it in medical terms, and offer medical solutions. Only physicians have the cultural authority to define the conditions that fall within the scope of medicine.

Physician authority is of relatively recent origin (Starr 1982). Nineteenth-century physicians were a heterogeneous group espousing a number of widely divergent medical ideologies. Most had little education or formal training. They plied their trade in a free market, unfettered by regulatory licensure and unaware of most of the scientific principles of modern medicine. Lacking anesthesia and antisepsis for most of the century, as well as blood transfusions and antibiotics, physicians' treatment outcomes were mixed. A vigorous campaign, orchestrated by the American Medical Association (AMA) with the help of the Carnegie Foundation and government legislatures, established allopathic medicine as the dominant ideology of the twentieth century.

In the process, the AMA increased the admission standards, length, and scientific rigor of medical education while decreasing the number of programs. Their emphasis on new scientific knowledge and improved outcomes convinced the public of the legitimate complexity and value of medicine and of the ethical, altruistic aims of the occupation. As a result, allopathic physicians won regulatory licensure under peer control in the early part of the twentieth century. The quacks and other "irregulars" were, for the most part, conquered. This "Great Trade" gave organized medicine autonomy and authority. In exchange the public was promised physicians who would serve their health care needs with the most effective medical treatments available, based on the latest scientific research.

The medical profession's mandate is to maximize the health and physical functioning of the population. As discussed in chapter 3, cosmetic surgery has been controversial among physicians because it entails placing patients at physical risk for mere appearance enhancement. Physicians who choose to use their considerable skills for such nonfunctional outcomes justify their decision in most cases in terms of the mental health of the patient. This justification, however, overlooks the influence of the changing structural dimensions of the political economy of medicine, dimensions that also encourage physicians to take up cosmetic surgery. This chapter discusses these structural dimensions. They include (1) the overall increase in the number of physicians, particularly surgical specialists; (2) the changing demand for some traditional surgical procedures; (3) the Federal Trade Commission (FTC) and AMA policies to promote "free trade" within the profession of medicine; (4) the breakdown of informal controls over cosmetic surgery, including restricted access to training, hospital privileges, and patients; and (5) the growth of managed care. The chapter concludes with a discussion of the efforts of the specialists most closely associated with cosmetic surgery, board-certified plastic surgeons, to maintain a separate identity and an elite image in the face of the changing political economy of medicine and encroachment by other physicians.

The Increasing Supply and Specialization of Physicians

Medicine has been in a continual state of change throughout the twentieth century. The educational reforms and consolidation of physician authority in the first quarter led to a decline in the number of physicians relative to the size of the population by mid-century. At the same time, the per capita demand for physicians increased. This demand was stimulated by both the efficacy of new therapies and the spread of private medical insurance as a worker benefit. The demand intensified in the mid-1960s when the publicly funded Medicare and Medicaid insurance programs opened the door to subsidized health care for the elderly and poor. There did not seem to be enough physicians to meet the health care demands of the rapidly growing population.

In response to widespread public concern about a doctor shortage, the federal government funded a massive increase in the number and size of medical schools between 1965 and 1980; this doubled the annual number of graduates (Starr 1982, 421). The government also opened the door to foreign medical school graduates. As a result, by 1975, 35 percent of newly licensed physicians were graduates of foreign medical schools, not counting those from Canada (Bureau of the Census 1990, 101). The impact of these two policies was substantial. By 1980 there were 211 physicians for every 100,000 people, compared to 155 in 1965 (Bureau of the Census 1984, 102). Concern about too many physicians replaced concern about too few (Department of Health and Human Services 1980). Although medical school enrollments have been reduced since 1982 (Marder et al. 1988, 28) and the influx of foreign medical school graduates has been curtailed, the momentum of the previous medical school expansion pushed the number of medical doctors to 737,764 and the number of osteopathic doctors to 37,300, yielding a combined ratio of 291 per 100,000 by 1996 (Bureau of the Census 1998, 129). Another 170,000 are in training (*American Medical News* 1997).

The increased supply of physicians intensified existing financial and technological pressures on physicians to specialize within medicine. Physicians are a far less homogeneous occupation than in 1970 when 17 percent of medical doctors were general practitioners and 9 percent were general surgeons (Randolph 1997, 21–22). The 71 percent decrease in general practitioners between 1970 and 1996 has been somewhat offset by the growth of the new primary care specialty of family practice after 1975. Nevertheless, in 1996 only 11 percent of active medical doctors reported a general or family practice and only 5 percent reported being general surgeons. The rest work in more specialized areas, none of which account for more than 6 percent of medical doctors, except for internal medicine (17 percent) and pediatrics

(7 percent). A few specialties, like public health, forensic pathology, and plastic surgery, each contain less than 1 percent of all practicing medical doctors.

Specialties divide medical practice into twenty-four board-certified areas recognized by the American Board of Medical Specialties (ABMS). They range from allergy and immunology to urology. They include older, well-established specialties like the American Board of Ophthalmology, the first specialty board established in 1917; the American Board of Otolaryngology, the second, established in 1924; and the American Board of Plastic Surgery, an ABMS member since 1941. They also include new specialties like emergency medicine and medical genetics. The ABMS estimates that at least 85 percent of practicing physicians are certified by ABMS member boards (Stevens 1999). All ABMS boards require additional years of education and practice experience, as well as evidence of mastery of the specialized area knowledge on comprehensive written and oral examinations. Many offer additional certification in "subspecialties." For example, obstetrics and gynecology has certificates of special qualifications in gynecologic oncology, maternal and fetal medicine, and reproductive endocrinology. Some, such as internal medicine, have numerous official subspecialties, while others, such as plastic surgery, have only one (i.e., hand surgery). The ABMS also grants certificates of added qualifications that are conceptually an emphasis within the broader specialty, rather than a subspecialization within a narrower field.

At least 100 additional self-designated boards are not members of the ABMS (Gradinger 1995). Approximately 10 of these involve some plastic surgery techniques. These boards also set standards of training and certify competence, although their requirements vary. The American Board of Facial Plastic and Reconstructive Surgery, for example, requires that all applicants already be certified by either the American Board of Plastic Surgery or the American Board of Otolaryngology, both members of the ABMS. The vast majority are certified by the latter board, which reports that more than one-quarter of its certifying examination is devoted to plastic surgery (Page 1989a, 49). In contrast, the American Board of Cosmetic Surgery offers both area-specific certification in body and extremity, dermatologic, and facial cosmetic surgery and general certification in all areas. Like the American Board of Facial Plastic and Reconstructive Surgery, this board will certify applicants who are already certified in an "equivalent specialty" by an ABMS member board and have additional experience in cosmetic surgery. Unlike the American Board of Facial Plastic and Reconstructive Surgery, the American Board of Cosmetic Surgery will recognize board certification in other areas as well, if they have some surgical training and successfully complete a general written examination and a specific oral examination in each area for which certification is sought. Some members are osteopathic physicians.

Some of these self-designated boards may be recognized eventually by the ABMS, following the path of others in the past. Specialization is an ongoing process. New specialty boards and subspecialties within existing board areas continuously emerge and further subdivide medical practice. General radiology, for example, has declined while diagnostic radiology and radiation oncology have grown. Sociologists argue that the segmentation of medicine created by specialization makes physicians more interdependent and, consequently, reduces competition and fosters greater professional cohesion (Starr 1982, 18, 111). This is not always the case. Occasionally the evolving division of labor creates territorial disputes, as is the case in hand surgery, an official subspecialty of orthopedic surgery, general surgery, and plastic surgery. Intense territorial disputes also exist in cosmetic surgery, an unofficial self-designated subspecialty within many specialties.

Several state medical licensure boards already recognize certification by the American Board of Facial Plastic and Reconstructive Surgery as "substantially equivalent," for surgery of the head and neck, to that of the American Board of Plastic Surgery, much to the dismay of the latter (Neale 1996). The American Board of Plastic Surgery also continues to resist the intensifying efforts of the American Board of Otolaryngology to establish either a separate certificate of added qualifications in facial plastic reconstructive surgery or a joint subspecialty certificate in plastic surgery within the head and neck. Support for the plastic surgeons' defensive position among other ABMS member boards is eroding and some type of horizontal pathway to formal certification of otolaryngologists in aesthetic facial plastic surgery is likely, despite plastic surgeons' opposition to encroachment into their occupational territory.

Plastic surgeons' occupational territory is highly vulnerable to invasion. They are few in number. Only about five thousand have been board certified in plastic surgery, and only forty-eight hundred, less than 1 percent of all physicians, are in active practice in the United States (American Society of Plastic and Reconstructive Surgeons, 1999, personal communication). Plastic surgery is the only surgical disci-

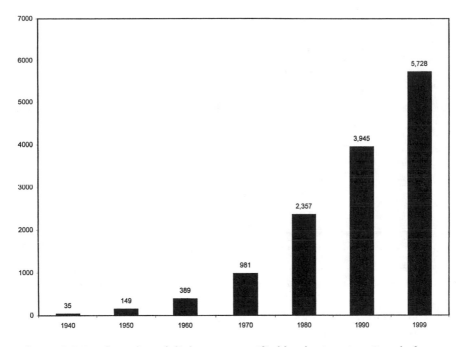

Figure 4.1. Total number of diplomates certified by the American Board of Plastic Surgery.

Note: The data include some plastic surgeons who are no longer in practice. For example, in 1999 approximately 4,800 were in active practice.

Source: American Board of Plastic Surgery, 1999, unpublished statistics.

pline without anatomic boundaries. These specialists have staked out the skin and its contents as their domain, overlapping other specialties' anatomic territorial claims. According to the 1996 president of the American Society of Plastic and Reconstructive Surgeons (ASPRS), which represents approximately 97 percent of all board-certified plastic surgeons, the specialty's "specialty" is really a philosophical commitment to surgical innovation, refinement, and excellence (Brody 1996a). Plastic surgeons have been on the cutting edge of replantation, organ transplantation, hand, burn, maxillofacial, and craniofacial surgery, as well as cosmetic surgery. But, defending occupational boundaries based on claims of greater surgical skill has proven to be difficult on almost all fronts. The lack of outcome data to support their claims has not helped (Krizek and Ketch 1994).

Otolaryngologists and other physicians have encroached plastic surgeons' territory on the cosmetic front at the same time orthopedic surgeons, general surgeons, oral surgeons, and others have invaded other fronts. The increased interspecialty competition has been exacerbated by increased intraspecialty competition. Figure 4.1 shows the rapid increase in the number of board-certified plastic surgeons in the last six decades. As a result of the specialty's own growth, as well as the increased number of other physicians attracted to cosmetic surgery, the number of medical doctors who self-designate their primary area of practice as plastic surgery has almost quadrupled between 1970 and 1996 (see table 4.1). Yet, only 62 percent report board certification in this area (Randolph 1997, 65). More than one-fifth are not certified by any ABMS-recognized board and another 16 percent are certified by a different ABMS-recognized board. Some of these physicians are in the process of fulfilling the requirements for board certification in plastic surgery. Others who are not board certified in plastic surgery limit themselves to cosmetic procedures that fall within their own specialty's training, such as otolaryngology, dermatology, or ophthalmology. Still others, including general surgeons, otolaryngologists, dermatologists, and ophthalmologists, branch out and incorporate additional cosmetic procedures into their practice, even to the point of becoming primarily cosmetic surgeons. This trend is evident in the advertisements discussed in chapter 6.

Most cosmetic surgery is performed by plastic surgeons, otolaryngologists, general surgeons, dermatologists, and ophthalmologists. Few practitioners specialize in only cosmetic surgery. Those who do usually join some related professional organization, other than the

Table 4.1 Physicians by Selected Self-Designated Specialties, 1970– 1996.

	1970	1980	1990	1996	1970–1996 % CHANGE
Plastic Surgery	1,600	2,980	4,590	5,896	269
Otolaryngology	5,409	6,553	8,138	9,028	67
Ophthalmology	9,927	12,974	16,073	17,777	79
Dermatology	4,003	5,660	7,557	8,854	121
All Physicians	334,028	467,679	615,421	737,764	121

Note: The data in this table refer to federal and nonfederal medical doctors; osteopathic physicians, who number more than 43,000 (American Osteopathic Association 1999), are not included.
Source: Lillian Randolph, *Physician Characteristics and Distribution in the U.S..* (Chicago: American Medical Association, 1997–1998).

ASPRS and the American Society for Aesthetic Plastic Surgery which admit only board-certified plastic surgeons. These professional specialty organizations assist in the development of residency training, sponsor postgraduate training programs, provide members with access to clinical practice, and give political and other information of interest to the specialty in journals, meetings, continuing education programs, and newsletters. The organizations provide a unified voice to speak on behalf of the members to government administrators and legislators, the public, and other medical organizations. They also offer a referral service for prospective patients.

Board-certified ophthalmologists founded the American Society of Ophthalmic Plastic and Reconstructive Surgery in 1969. This subspecialty organization of approximately 300 members sponsors a professional journal, educational symposia, and fellowship training in cosmetic and reconstructive procedures (American Society of Ophthalmic Plastic and Reconstructive Surgery 1997). Board-certified otolaryngologists similarly founded the American Academy of Facial Plastic and Reconstructive Surgery in 1964. Membership in the academy has grown from less than 1,000 in 1970 to between 2,700 and 3,000 in the 1990s (American Academy of Facial Plastic and Reconstructive Surgery, 1997, personal communication). In 1986 they established the American Board of Facial Plastic and Reconstructive Surgery, which has certified about 400 practitioners since 1991, including a few plastic surgeons (American Board of Facial Plastic and Reconstructive Surgery, 1997, personal communication). Their certification, however, is not recognized by the ABMS.

Otolaryngologists who do cosmetic procedures in other areas of the body as well as in the head and neck region, along with physicians from other backgrounds, such as dermatology, founded in 1969 the multi-specialty American Association of Cosmetic Surgeons, which did not begin recruiting members until 1974 when the American Society for Aesthetic Plastic Surgery refused to admit them (Williams et al. 1978). This organization gave birth to the American Board of Cosmetic Surgery in 1979 (to offer certification) and the American Academy of Cosmetic Surgery in 1985 (House 1989a, 259, 283). By mid-1997, 325 physicians were certified by this board (American Board of Cosmetic Surgery, 1997, personal communication); membership in the academy, which does not require board certification, was approximately 1,100 (American Academy of Cosmetic Surgery, 1997, personal communication). This certification also is not recognized by the ABMS.

The increased competition for patients from physicians trained outside plastic surgery has led to the intense turf battle discussed in chapter 5. Concern is nearly as great about the growing intraspecialty competition. There was 1 board-certified plastic surgeon for every 250,000 Americans in 1974, and the ASPRS believed that more were needed (Hait 1994, 67A). Residency programs expanded rapidly, graduating almost 300 annually in the mid-1970s. By 1995 there was 1 plastic surgeon for every 56,600 people in the United States, compared to 1 for every 350,000 in the United Kingdom (*Plastic Surgery News* 1995d). The Royal College of Surgeons maintains that 1 per 125,000 would be ideal. Editorials and letters to the editor in *Plastic and Reconstructive Surgery* and *Plastic Surgery News* in the 1980s and 1990s complain about the impact of the oversupply on the specialty. The authors suggest that the shrinking ratio is pushing plastic surgeons into cosmetic surgery and causing a few to adopt unethical practices to stimulate demand and reduce competition.

The annual number of physicians completing plastic surgery residencies has been held constant at about 200 to 220 since the early 1990s because of the widespread concern about oversupply. If plastic surgery residency programs continue to graduate that many, the number practicing will double by the year 2040. The ratio would then be reduced to 1 plastic surgeon for every 38,461 people (*Plastic Surgery News* 1994e). If the number of graduates were reduced by 40 percent, as advocated by some leaders, the ratio would still rise to 1 for every 50,000 people by 2010 because the older, retiring cohorts during this period will be much smaller in number than the cohorts entering practice. After 2010 the number in retiring cohorts would approximately equal the number in entering cohorts, if reduced by 40 percent, and the ratio would decline to about the same level as in 1995.

The prospect of continued growth in the number of trained plastic surgeons is viewed with alarm by most board-certified plastic surgeons. The ASPRS designated the oversupply of plastic surgeons and the corresponding increased competition for patients as the organization's number one priority in 1997 (*Plastic Surgery News* 1996c). In spite of the increasing number of board-certified plastic surgeons, the total number of reconstructive procedures they reported in 1994 was 13 percent less than in 1992 (*Plastic Surgery News* 1995e). Cosmetic procedures also declined overall by 5 percent over the two years following the negative publicity surrounding the (Food and Drug Administration) FDA's imposed moratorium on silicone breast implants.

Dramatic increases in breast implant removals and upper arm lifts and moderate increases in saline breast augmentations and liposuction did not offset substantial declines in nose modifications, chemical peels, and eye lifts. The ASPRS study projected that if residencies were not substantially reduced, the average number of procedures per surgeon would fall by more than one-third. This decline would occur even if the per capita number of cosmetic procedures increased, as expected, due to the anticipated aging of the population and increasing affluence. A reduction in the number of plastic surgery residency graduates by about one-third was proposed (Ruberg 1994) and remains under debate at this time. This proposal would maintain the availability of plastic surgery residents in hospitals by increasing all plastic surgery residency programs to three years.

Rapid increases in the number of cosmetic procedures since 1994 may have eased concerns about the oversupply of plastic surgeons somewhat. This increase was led by liposuction, breast augmentation, eyelid surgery, and breast implant removals. The total number of reconstructive procedures continues to decline, despite significant increases in breast reconstruction and breast reduction.

Changing Demand for Medical Procedures

Increases in the number of practicing plastic surgeons and otolaryngologists occurred as demand for some of their noncosmetic skills declined. Geographic regionalization of craniofacial surgery and burn treatment and the use of safety belts and shatterproof glass in automobiles reduced the need for plastic surgeons to function as local "trauma specialists" (Goldwyn 1977). Similarly, the decline in the number of births between 1960 and the late 1970s reduced the number of cleft palates and other congenital craniofacial deformities. Government programs that increased earlier access to medical care among the poor and elderly, together with innovations in radiation and chemotherapy, also decreased the incidence of large tumors and other disease-caused deformities that had been a part of the traditional domain of plastic surgery. Finally, organ transplants, an area where plastic surgeons helped to pioneer surgical techniques, have become primarily an immunological medical problem (Brody 1996a).

The declining demand for reconstructive procedures, despite an increasing number of plastic surgeons, creates a tight market. Only 7 percent have a purely reconstructive practice (Iverson 1997). Most, 59 percent, spend half or more of their time on cosmetic surgery. Cosmetic surgery allows these surgeons to maintain their highly refined surgical skills that are in less demand. At the same time, it provides them with healthy patients who have a lower risk of complications and gives them a fast turnover and an attractive economic reward.

Socioeconomic well-being emerged as a major concern among plastic surgeons in the late 1980s, exacerbating the impact of their increasing supply. Although their median net income was approximately double that of family practitioners and pediatricians, the increase in plastic surgeons' earnings failed to match the cost of living increase in 1988, a period when physicians as a whole had the highest increase in the sixty-one years that such data have been collected (Owens 1990). There were growing complaints that some established plastic surgeons deliberately create difficulties for younger plastic surgeons to protect their market (Gorney 1984, 121). A former ASPRS president argued that "to protect the public we would have to cut the numbers and raise the standards" (Gorney 1989a, 800–801), a policy that also would protect the economic interests of established plastic surgeons.

Demand for some traditional otolaryngology procedures, especially tonsillectomies, adenoidectomies, and surgical intervention in bacterial infections, declined after the introduction of antibiotics and the emergence of allergy specialists and the paramedical field of audiology (Bailey 1987). In the 1960s many otolaryngologists concentrated on correcting hearing problems, but demand dwindled as the backlog of potential patients received treatment. In response, otolaryngologists turned to head and neck cancer surgery in the 1970s. This led to an interest and training in aesthetic results and, ultimately, cosmetic surgery (Regan 1985). Facelifts, chin and nose modifications, ear pinning, and even eye lifts became part of many otolaryngologists' repertoires. The president of the otolaryngologists' American Society of Head and Neck Surgery in the late 1980s expressed fear that new members of his specialty were being pushed into cosmetic surgery because of the limited number of head and neck cancers (Lore 1988). He also advocated reducing the number of residencies in his specialty, a policy that would protect the economic interests of established otolaryngologists as well.

Dermatology also has undergone considerable change over the last forty years (Chrisman 1989). Starting in the late 1950s, dermatologists began adding surgical procedures such as dermabrasion and hair trans plants. The 1960s and 1970s brought Mohs' surgery for skin cancers. A close liaison with otolaryngologists introduced advanced plastic techniques to treat wounds resulting from skin cancer removal. By the late 1970s some dermatologists were doing scalp reductions and using flaps for hair replacement. At the same time that dermatology added surgical techniques to its repertoire, other traditional nonsurgical problems—venereal diseases, collagen diseases, pediatric dermatology, and allergies—were absorbed by other specialties. By the 1990s residencies in dermatology included facelifts, liposuction, and lipo-injection as well as hair replacement.

Free Trade within Medicine

Supply and demand factors help to explain why plastic surgeons and otolaryngologists, both of whom have training in plastic and reconstructive techniques, have taken up cosmetic surgery. To understand the entry of other kinds of physicians into cosmetic surgery, additional structural factors must be considered. One is the nature of medical licensure. In spite of the specialties that divide the actual practice of members of the profession, medical licensure encompasses all areas of medicine. Although the AMA promotes graduate medical education, the organization opposes the idea of specialty licenses and a hierarchical division of labor among physicians based on specialty training. Consequently, the relationships between primary practitioners and specialists and among specialists remain amorphous.

Contrary to popular belief, a medical license contains no restrictions against physicians doing cosmetic or any other surgical or medical procedures, regardless of training or specialty certification (Courtiss 1986). Moreover, physicians can designate themselves as specialists without obtaining approval from the certifying board in that specialty area (Reade and Ratzan 1987, 1318). Although such self-designated specialists and those certified by boards not recognized by the ABMS often are denied hospital privileges for this work, a 1984 AMA policy says that hospital privileges should be granted on the basis of training and experience and that board certification is not the only measure. This policy deliberately omits certification by an ABMS-approved board as a criterion and allows physicians to argue that they have equivalent training and experience. The AMA also rejects the idea that board certification should be the sole criterion for participation in managed care plans.

Opening the door to other physicians to work as plastic surgeons

threatens the tenuous claims of the specialty to greater skill. Consequently, the American Board of Plastic Surgery and its sister organization, the ASPRS, object strenuously to state medical boards formally
recognizing the training of physicians such as otolaryngologists certified by the American Board of Facial Plastic and Reconstructive Surgery as "substantially equivalent" to their own. These two organizations
similarly object to "certificates of added qualifications" in facial plastic
surgery, certificates that are not under the control of the American
Board of Plastic Surgery. Plastic surgeons also fear that the public will
assume that they are equivalent to general surgeons and that the "facial plastic surgeons" and the "cosmetic surgeons" are the true specialists in aesthetic surgery. In contrast, otolaryngologists and other
specialists who do cosmetic surgery vehemently argue that they have
the expertise and the legal right to offer cosmetic procedures.

The FTC also endorses free trade in medicine. The commission
filed twenty-seven health care antitrust cases between the mid-1970s
and the mid-1980s (Costillo 1985). The commission successfully challenged professional associations' attempts to restrict advertising and
access to legally qualified practitioners. As part of this campaign the
FTC subpoenaed ASPRS records in 1976 and subsequently claimed
that the ASPRS's use of board certification as a criterion for membership and patient referral violated the antitrust laws (Williams et al.
1978). The ASPRS assessed its members four hundred dollars each and
spent half a million dollars to defend itself in negotiations that spanned
three and one-half years (Hait 1994, 73A). The FTC eventually ceased
to pursue its complaint in 1980. Although the commission offered no
explanation for its decision, it may have concluded that board certification no longer unfairly restrained the practice of medicine after it
pressured the AMA into signing a decree allowing doctors to advertise. Moreover, it may not have thought that there was sufficient evidence linking the society to its members' local efforts to restrain the
trade of other physicians (Oliver 1989). Despite its policy to downplay
the significance of certification by an ABMS board, the FTC did express concern about physicians whose formal training and experience
is unrelated to the medical services they offer and whose claims about
expertise and risks may be deceptive (*Plastic Surgery News* 1990d).
Like the AMA, however, the commission does not regard certification
by an ABMS board as the only measure of a physician's qualifications.
Instead, the FTC relies on state medical boards to evaluate a physician's
qualifications.

Breakdown of Informal Controls over Cosmetic Surgery

Regulation of specialty practice is left to the informal peer controls exerted in selection for residency programs, permission to use hospital facilities, referral of patients between colleagues, and the prospect of licensure revocation and increased vulnerability in malpractice litigation for not adhering to the prevailing standards of medical practice. These informal regulatory processes, however, no longer deter physicians who lack formal training or board certification in plastic and reconstructive surgery from doing cosmetic surgery.

Access to Training

Through the 1960s, residency programs in plastic surgery provided little or no training in cosmetic surgery and few surgeons who did aesthetic procedures were willing to share their knowledge (Hait 1994, 63A). Many residency programs continue to focus primarily on reconstructive work, even though much of plastic surgeons' work is cosmetic (Krizek and Ketch 1994, 87). Cosmetic surgery fundamentally rests on techniques developed for reconstructive work, but the particular aims of cosmetic surgery have created unique problems, challenges, and procedures.

To educate themselves, as well as others, a small group founded the American Society for Aesthetic Plastic Surgeons in 1967 to have an opportunity to share information about cosmetic surgery. Several others organized what has since become the Annual Symposium on Cosmetic Surgery (*Plastic Surgery News* 1994b). Fifty physicians attended the first in 1966. Applications increased as the popularity of cosmetic surgery expanded. The organizers now cap attendance at 450, but say they could easily fill a room of 750. The success of this "tell and show" format with live demonstrations spawned many others, most focused on a single procedure or set of procedures. As a result, new techniques quickly spread among practitioners. For example, few practicing physicians whose residencies were in the 1970s and 1980s were trained in liposuction or some of the other cosmetic procedures now in high demand. Most learn new procedures at weekend workshops and symposia sponsored by specialty associations such as the ASPRS, the American Academy of Facial Plastic and Reconstructive Surgery, and the American Academy of Cosmetic Surgery. The latter opens its programs to all licensed physicians, undermining the other two associations' control of access to training.

Hospital Privileges

Lack of hospital privileges no longer impedes physicians who want to do cosmetic surgery. Cosmetic surgery began to move out of hospitals in the 1970s, and 95 percent now takes place in doctors' offices and surgicenters (House 1989a, 117). Because board-certified plastic surgeons, otolaryngologists, ophthalmologists, and dermatologists led the relocation, office-based cosmetic surgery has become the accepted standard of practice, placing it out of sight of peers and eliminating the need to obtain hospital privileges.

Cosmetic surgery's move out of the hospital was fueled by patients' desire for lower costs and both patients' and physicians' desire for greater convenience. The savings have come at a great cost for a few patients. Patients have died because of a lack of adequate safety precautions, and others have had unnecessary complications (*Plastic Surgery News* 1993c). As discussed in chapter 8, the number of deaths and serious complications are unknown because office surgery is exempt from the reporting requirements that apply to hospitals and licensed surgicenters in all states except New Jersey and Florida. It is also exempt from mandatory accreditation requirements in every state except California. A 1992 Department of Health and Human Services inspection of 160 facilities run by plastic surgeons and other physicians in four states revealed that 131 were neither licensed nor accredited, including 7 of the 21 performing "high risk" procedures. Over half have no written medical emergency procedure; 80 percent have no life support or resuscitation equipment. Despite the risks, there is no regulation of office-based cosmetic surgery in almost all states. Any physician who can recruit patients can legally perform office-based cosmetic surgery.

Advertising

Lack of referrals from other physicians is no longer a serious obstacle to doing cosmetic surgery. In 1975 the U.S. Supreme Court ruled, in *Goldfarb v. Virginia State Bar,* that lawyers and other "learned professions" are not exempt from the Sherman Antitrust Act. As discussed in more detail in chapter 6, the FTC used this ruling to charge the AMA and two local medical societies with restraint of trade because of their bans on personal advertising by physicians (Avellone and Moore 1978). Over the vehement opposition of the ASPRS (Gorney 1989b) and to the dismay of the AMA (*American Medical News* 1977), the Supreme Court affirmed the FTC's position in 1982. As a result, cosmetic surgery became a blatantly commercial enterprise.

Paid advertisements, some with pictures that look like *Playboy* centerfolds, now reach out for consumers in the mail, Yellow Pages, newspapers, local magazines, airline magazines and on benches, buses, subways, billboards, symphony playbills, radio, television, and the Internet. In Southern California, where competition is intense, one physician was estimated to spend $750,000 on his annual multimedia campaign in the late 1980s (Gorney 1989b). Physicians also promote themselves through interviews with journalists, reporters, and talk show hosts and in newspaper columns, books, "educational seminars," and health fairs. These public relations endeavors provide exposure and an opportunity to expound on new techniques, safety, and social, economic, and psychological benefits and to give guidance on how to choose a physician, how to be a good candidate for cosmetic surgery, and financing. The content of these marketing strategies and the implications for the profession of medicine and health care are discussed in greater detail in chapters 6 and 7.

Corporatization of Health Care Delivery

Free trade in medicine and the breakdown of informal controls over cosmetic surgery make it possible for physicians who feel pressured by increased competition and declining demand for their noncosmetic services to take up cosmetic surgery. Many also view cosmetic surgery as a chance to escape the corporate transformation of the health care system. Cosmetic surgery is largely an out-of-pocket, fee-for-service business, devoid of third-party regulatory oversight and paperwork. Physicians who spend at least half their time on cosmetic surgery, about half of board-certified plastic surgeons (Iverson 1997) and 57 percent of the members of the American Academy of Cosmetic Surgery (1999), have more control over their work. They can be virtually independent practitioners at a time when corporatization is transforming most physicians into employees. In 1997, 59 percent of board-certified plastic surgeons were still solo practitioners, as were 66 percent of the members of the American Academy of Cosmetic Surgery, compared to only 19 percent of all medical doctors (Randolph 1997, 43).

Physicians who do cosmetic surgery are, nonetheless, vulnerable to the market forces driving corporatization. The proportion of board-certified plastic surgeons in solo practice has been falling rapidly in recent years. Moreover, 80 percent report contracts with managed care organizations (American Society of Plastic and Reconstructive Surgeons 1997). These contracts, however, contribute only 27 percent of their income. Six percent report that all their income is from cosmetic surgery; another one-third report that three-quarters of their income is from cosmetic surgery, even though only 26 percent spend three-quarters or more of their time on cosmetic surgery (Iverson 1997). Clearly, cosmetic surgery is the economic backbone of many practices. It amounts to 40 percent of the procedures done by a typical board-certified plastic surgeon (*Plastic Surgery News* 1995f).

Some practitioners fear that cosmetic surgery will not remain in the fee-for-service domain. Instead, they speculate that it may be integrated as a for-profit component of managed care programs in the future (Pearl et al. 1997). Even if cosmetic surgery remains a fee-for-service enterprise, physicians who want to continue to do reconstructive work must look increasingly to managed care programs for patients. The ASPRS began a program called Managing Your Health Care Environment in 1994 to help plastic surgeons adapt to the changing structure of health care delivery (Hait 1994, 90A). When some complained that they were being shut out of managed care programs, the ASPRS responded with *A Practical Guide to Marketing Your Plastic Surgery Services to Managed Care* in 1996 to help members gain entry to managed care programs. The ASPRS now targets managed care organizations as part of its larger, long-standing public relations campaign on behalf of plastic surgeons. The organization sent twenty-five hundred copies of both *Procedures in Plastic Surgery*, which provides clinical information on indications, selection criteria, and outcome expectations for plastic surgeons, and *Plastic Surgeons: A Delineation of Qualifications for Clinical Privileges* to managed care administrators in 1994 (*Plastic Surgery News* 1995c).

Marketing the Specialty
and the Specialists

The FTC's pursuit of professional associations' bans on advertising in the 1970s was viewed as a calamity by physician leaders, particularly in plastic surgery. They claimed that the FTC's desire to decrease the cost of medical services by increasing competition between practitioners would jeopardize the public's health. Medical care, they argued, is more complex than other goods and services. Lacking medical knowledge, consumers had to depend on professional control over access to specialty training and hospital privileges and, most importantly, peer referral to protect them from exploitation by unscrupulous practitioners. Allowing physicians to advertise directly to the public undermines this traditional self-regulatory system. Combined with the shift to an increasing amount of out-of-hospital surgery and the growth of plastic surgery training in other specialties, the policy ended plastic surgeons' virtual monopoly over most types of cosmetic surgery.

The External Public Relations Campaign

Responding to the FTC, the outgoing president of the ASPRS in 1978 claimed, "We are not going to become marketers—or advertisers—but we shall attempt to educate the public to protect itself" (Peterson 1978). His overall vision of the role of advertising in medicine proved to be myopic; a few physicians began to advertise immediately. Not surprisingly, cosmetic surgery, the most elective of all surgical procedures, led the medical marketing revolution. Some of the advertisements are subdued announcements of procedures offered; others are in dubious taste, as discussed in chapter 6. At least one physician thought that a "BOOBS" license plate would attract patients.

At first few members of the ASPRS participated in paid advertising. They relied on their professional association to conduct a public relations campaign on their behalf. The ASPRS had begun some public relations efforts in the 1950s and 1960s designed to promote the specialty and inform the public about plastic surgery innovations in an organized way. The new campaign, in contrast, aggressively reached out to the public through the media to defend and enhance the separate identity and elite image of the specialty. The public relations firm hired in 1976 was directed to prepare feature stories on plastic surgery that emphasized the need for a board-certified plastic surgeon and to ensure that at least one such feature appeared every month in a women's magazine or on the broadcast media (Williams et al. 1978, 20). Twelve articles were prepared in the first year.

The ASPRS's invigorated public relations campaign grew bolder in promoting the external image of the specialty. The message was three-fold: "We are," "We care," and "We dare to lead" or, more generally, "Doing what others do—best!" (Peterson 1977). They chose California as the test site because individual physician advertisements were most prolific there. The ASPRS placed announcements offering free copies of a booklet, *How to Shop for a Qualified Surgeon*, in fifteen newspapers and on radio (Goin 1978). The society also issued news releases to all newspapers, magazines, and television stations in the state, resulting in additional free, favorable coverage of the society's campaign to "educate" the public. The campaign resulted in over fourteen hundred requests for the booklets. The ASPRS also trained members of its Speakers Bureau about how to respond to interviewers. Individual self-promotion was discouraged. When asked about cosmetic surgery, they were told to "bridge" the discussion to reconstructive surgery, the number of board-certified plastic surgeons, the availability of cosmetic services to ordinary people in the middle class, and the psychological importance of body image (*Plastic Surgery News* 1977). After the ASPRS gained more experience with media interviews that produced results other than what they wanted, the society warned plastic surgeons to stick to their own agenda, stay serious and scientific, and never become too comfortable with a reporter. Moreover, the society told members to avoid answering any questions about money, especially regarding the surgeon's own earnings (*Plastic Surgery News* 1993e).

Marketing became the major priority of the 1981–1982 ASPRS president, William Porterfield, a choice that proved to be highly controversial at the time. Some applauded him for turning the ASPRS into a business organization; others condemned him for merchandising the proud specialty (Hait 1994, 76A–77A). The marketing consultant he hired made a series of recommendations, ranging from developing a new logo and a system for financing patients' cosmetic surgery to a public information program. The latter included not only an expansion of the public relations underway, but also the development of a series of brochures on cosmetic procedures, brochures that could be given to prospective patients for consideration during a consultation.

The ASPRS adopted eight general themes for the public information program (Hugo 1982a):

- Plastic and reconstructive surgeons are highly trained specialists with at least two additional years of residency after a minimum of three years of general surgery.
- They are committed to the constant exchange of information on

developments by peers and required to participate in continuing education.

- They treat a wide range of deformities, congenital, traumatic, cancerous, and aging, and are responsible for many innovations in surgery.
- They are committed to excellent and ethical care and they monitor each other.
- Plastic surgery can enhance the quality of life for those who undergo it for personal, professional, physical, or social reasons.
- Plastic surgeons counsel patients on the potential and limitations to make sure they have realistic expectations.
- The ASPRS offers a Patient Referral Service. If patients do not use this service, they should make sure that their physicians are board-certified in plastic and reconstructive surgery and have hospital privileges in plastic surgery.
- The public must be informed about the value and efficacy of procedures, prostheses, and materials.

When the society assessed members $650 each to fund the public education program, a few resigned in protest against the unabashed marketing. In spite of the initial opposition, a decade later most of the consultant's recommendations were in place and periodic assessments have been levied to pay for the marketing efforts.

The society also revived a science writers symposium that had proven successful at national meetings in 1965 and 1970, started a new program to bring interesting reconstructive cases to the attention of the media, and began to monitor media coverage. The latter revealed the immediate, successful impact of the various public relations programs; the society was mentioned in 250 press clips in June 1982, almost double the 137 in the previous January (Hugo 1982b). The society was similarly successful with a mail outreach offer to broadcast media; more than 320 television and radio station program directors requested interviews with plastic surgeons.

The patient education brochures also were immediately successful. By the mid-1980s the society grossed over $1 million a year from their sale to members, who found, as the marketing consultant predicted, that prospective patients used them at home to decide to have these elective procedures (Hait 1994, 82A). They remain a lucrative source of income for the ASPRS. More members turned to the ASPRS for additional help with "practice enhancement," a euphemistic term for marketing strategies such as the brochures. No longer did the majority of plastic surgeons believe that the traditional marketing strategy of "ability, availability, and affability" was sufficient to attract patients.

The ASPRS abandoned a 1985 national advertising campaign that focused only on informing the public about the society. Members complained that these paid institutional ads did not bring in patients. Instead, the society combined its institutional advertising with other projects and began to sponsor seminars and workshops for members on how to market their individual practices (*Plastic Surgery News* 1985). When the scope of its marketing activities became too unwieldy for a committee to manage in 1986, the society established a separate marketing department to oversee its programs, products, and services as well as help members market their own practices (*Plastic Surgery News* 1986a). The society's news publication began to accept advertisements from marketing firms soliciting members' business with advertisements offering "A Starter Kit for the New Practice or the Practice New to Marketing," "Practice Expansion through Marketing Auxiliary Services," and "From Yellow Pages to Infomercials."

The number and types of marketing products and services available continued to expand (*Plastic Surgery News* 1987d). The society commissioned a short film, *Eye of the Beholder*, and a public education slide show that members could use for local seminars. The society developed the *Plastic Surgery Newsletter*, a quarterly that can be personalized with a physician's own name and photo and used to keep in contact with prospective and former patients and mailed to new prospects. The society set up an automated toll-free national referral service after a test in Kansas City produced 300 calls in response to two print advertisements and a televised public service announcement about the number (*Plastic Surgery News* 1986b). Adding a live operator the following year increased the number of the contacts by 25 percent (*Plastic Surgery News* 1987e). By 1994 the referral number, redefined as the "Plastic Surgery Information Service," logged an average of 6,600 calls a month (*Plastic Surgery News* 1995a). More than one-third of the callers sought referrals. The society published a commercially available book, *ASPRS' Guide to Cosmetic Surgery* in 1992, which discusses who is a good candidate for cosmetic surgery, the nature of the procedures available, and risks involved as well as advice about appropriate motivations and realistic expectations and, of course, how to choose a qualified surgeon.

Even as the ASPRS involvement in marketing grew rapidly, members continued to debate the issues involved. At a 1986 conference on strategies to help members develop marketing programs, participants debated whether it was appropriate for the society to use marketing to try to increase the demand for cosmetic surgery (*Plastic Surgery News* 1986c). Practicing plastic surgeons wrote to their journal and *Plastic Surgery News* to protest the trend. Typical of these letters to the editor was the view that marketing would undermine the profession. As one said, "The assertion that physicians must try to sell their practices is anathema to most legitimate plastic surgeons, who are in the profession to help people and not to fill a garage with Rolls Royces. . . . We, as plastic surgeons, are here to reconstruct the burned, the maimed and the cancer patient. The whole thrust of so-called 'marketing firms'—which are nothing more than advertising agencies—is toward the almighty dollar" (*Plastic Surgery News* 1989a, 12). A former president of the ASPRS worried that as a result of advertising, "People are being sold surgery that they don't need, that the surgeon is not thoroughly comfortable or familiar with, but he's got to do it to stay ahead" (*Plastic Surgery News* 1994c, 2–3).

Despite doomsday predictions only a decade earlier about the perils of marketing, by 1987 the ASPRS boasted to members that it had "harnessed" the power of the press (*Plastic Surgery News* 1987b). Clearly, the ASPRS was on the cutting edge of medical advertising. Using money collected in another assessment of members, the ASPRS responded aggressively to articles written under the influence of the fledgling public relations efforts of the American Academy of Facial Plastic and Reconstructive Surgery and the American Academy of Cosmetic Surgery because the society believed that the articles confused the public about who is best qualified to perform cosmetic surgery. The ASPRS communications staff personally visited key editors, writers, and producers to discuss their coverage of cosmetic surgery. The society also moved preemptively. It supplied radio stations with prerecorded messages about plastic surgery trends and issues and increased the training of regional media spokespersons. It also stepped up efforts to expose the media to its annual meetings and regional symposia. The media, particularly those targeted at women, received high priority because the society had evidence that media stories generate work for members. When two women's magazines, *Family Circle* and *Redbook*, published articles in the same month on cosmetic surgery, emphasizing the importance of finding a board-certified plastic surgeon, calls to the referral service increased 173 percent over the previous month (*Plastic Surgery News* 1988d). A subsequent study revealed that one 1990 cosmetic surgery article in *Family Circle* led 1,821 readers to call the toll-free number listed within six weeks (*Plastic Surgery News* 1990c). Individual physicians also recognize the value of cosmetic surgery articles in trusted magazines; some give prospective patients copies of them.

The ASPRS discovered that the media are interested in statistics about the number of cosmetic procedures and about costs. Only the ASPRS collected such information in the 1980s. Even though the members' response rate was only 15 percent in 1986, the society held three regional press conferences to release these data, and reporters from more than forty major newspapers, magazines, and radio and television stations attended (*Plastic Surgery News* 1987f). Additional press kits were mailed nationwide. Numerous reports on the rapid growth of cosmetic surgery followed. The society added a patient survey and a public survey to gather additional information to feed to the media. By carefully timing the release of these "newsworthy" data, the society discovered that it could generate year-long press coverage. Since 1992 the society has contracted for scientific sampling to provide better quality data. The American Academy of Facial Plastic and Reconstructive Surgery began to collect and release similar information after the success of the ASPRS's efforts, as did the American Society for Aesthetic Plastic Surgery, the sister organization of the ASPRS, and the American Academy of Cosmetic Surgery.

The ASPRS tried other creative marketing approaches in the late 1980s. The ASPRS sponsored three closed-circuit teleconferences in a talk-show format designed to help the public learn about cosmetic surgery and meet local plastic surgeons (*Plastic Surgery News* 1988a). These programs—"Minimizing the Effects of Aging," "Changing the Family 'Profile,'" and "Contouring the Body"—were sent via satellite to hospitals around the country where they were either shown live or taped for later use and reuse. Hospitals that ran advertisements in local newspapers attracted as many as 130 prospective patients to their individual screenings. Local ASPRS members were present to answer questions and meet with prospective patients and reporters after the show. The ASPRS teamed up with *Vogue* to hold a series of women's health and beauty workshops in department stores throughout the country (*Plastic Surgery News* 1988b). Plastic surgeons spoke and provided brochures and information on the society's referral service to the estimated 1,500 women who attended the various programs. Video news releases on plastic surgery in general and on specific cosmetic procedures, such as fat injection and liposuction, were distributed to cable television stations and generated 470 cable casts within a year; they were used by 8 commercial stations as well (*Plastic Surgery News* 1989b). A two-part video news release was produced in conjunction with the 1988 ASPRS scientific meeting, along with audiotapes for radio stations. Both proved effective; at least 154 television stations aired one or both parts of the video tapes and 398 radio stations aired the audiotapes. The society subsequently established the Plastic Surgery Network News to supply one-minute air spots. It also continues to produce audio and video news releases in conjunction with its annual meeting and to distribute some two thousand press kits of newsworthy information in advance, along with an invitation to the meeting.

Other associations of physicians who do cosmetic surgery have developed public relations campaigns. They have established national information-and-referral telephone numbers, offered spokespersons, worked with media reporters, developed materials to distribute to prospective patients, and issued press releases on innovations, as well as statistics on their number of procedures, costs, and the like. Nevertheless, the ASPRS public relations efforts have been much larger in scope and have succeeded in placing the ASPRS as the dominant source of information about cosmetic surgery. In 1990 the ASPRS was mentioned in 1,277 media reports compared to only 206 mentions of other organizations involved with cosmetic surgery (*Plastic Surgery News* 1991b). The ASPRS's statistics on procedures appeared in 852 reports compared to only 34 reports that mention other organizations' statistics. Most importantly, in the view of its members, the ASPRS referral service number was listed in 325 reports compared to only 41 mentions of the other organizations' referral services. The ASPRS's quick adaptation to the changing political economy of medicine allowed it to continue to dominate the market for cosmetic surgery.

The FDA and the Breast Implant Crisis

Physicians involved in cosmetic surgery faced a public relations problem when scientists at the Food and Drug Administration (FDA) in late 1990 leaked research results revealing that the polyurethane foam coating on two brands of breast implants broke down into known carcinogens. These devices, used in a minority of implant patients, were immediately withdrawn from the market by the manufacturer. The press coverage raised concern over the potential health risks of other types of breast implants and questions about whether the government and physicians had provided adequate protection for the public's health.

The content of the press coverage suggests that few realized that the FDA's authority did not encompass medical devices before 1976. The regulatory organization's oversight was then expanded in response to the exponential growth of implantable devices. As with new drugs, manufacturers now have to submit research evidence that a medical device is both safe and effective. Breast implants, however, were already in use before 1976 and were classified as needing only compliance with "performance standards." This is analogous to requiring the manufacturer of an EKG machine to provide evidence that it is free from shock hazard. Subsequent consumer complaints about breast implants, combined with a lack of scientific evidence of implant safety on file, led the FDA to require a premarket approval in mid-1988. The ASPRS filed numerous supportive documents, including the results of a patient satisfaction survey that found that 95 percent were satisfied with their implants and only 9 percent had considered having them removed. In the fall of 1991 the FDA warned manufacturers that the ongoing review of submitted data, including twenty-two crates of materials from Dow Corning, revealed major deficiencies in the type of documentation needed to assess safety (Hait 1994, 93A).

The breast-implant public relations problem suddenly became a full-fledged crisis. The ASPRS responded to the looming prospect that breast implants might be withdrawn from the market by assessing members $350 a year for three years to raise more than $4 million to address public policy issues and support research on breast implants. Additional donations poured into its political lobby organization, PlastyPAC. This was, according to the society, probably the most intense political effort on behalf of any medical specialty (*Plastic Surgery News* 1992c, insert). The society did the following:

- Retained three government relations firms to assist in communicating with policy makers;
- Established toll-free phone lines for members and patients;
- Organized grassroots letter-writing campaigns to congressmen;
- Established the Federal Action Support Team, a network of members to determine strategy;
- Organized a Washington "Fly-In" of about 200 plastic surgeons and

about 400 patients to tell legislators that breast implants are important for women's psychological well-being;

- Established a *Breast Implant Bulletin* to update members on developments;
- Sponsored newspaper advertisements, in five key congressional districts, that urged readers to call their congressional representatives and the FDA;
- Established the monthly *ASPRS Breast Implant Update* newsletter for patients;
- Hosted community forums with plastic surgeons, a psychologist, and patients to answer women's questions and attract media coverage;
- Established the Breast Implant Resource Center to respond to the needs of members involved in implant litigation;
- Sent members sample letters to sign and forward to Congress and the FDA.

In spite of the intense political pressure generated by these efforts, the ASPRS lost its battle. Its members also lost some credibility. In the fall of 1991 the FDA rescinded the voting rights of three plastic surgeons on its medical-device review panel because of concern about their potential conflict of interest. This direct affront to the authority and autonomy of physicians was challenged to no avail by the ASPRS, the AMA, and the American College of Surgeons. The remaining members of the panel concluded that the manufacturers' data were insufficient to evaluate the safety and efficacy of implants. Nevertheless, persuaded by the testimony of the ASPRS, AMA, American College of Surgeons, American College of Obstetrics and Gynecology, American Society for Aesthetic Plastic Surgery, and the American College of Radiology, the panel recommended that the devices remain available while manufacturers conduct scientific studies. To the horror of the ASPRS, the panel's recommendation was overruled by the FDA commissioner in January 1992. Responding to mounting public concern, fueled by media coverage of the increasing number of lawsuits claiming that implants cause autoimmune and other types of diseases and multimillion dollar awards against breast implant manufacturers, the commissioner announced a moratorium on silicone-gel breast implants for cosmetic purposes, unless they were part of a clinical research protocol. This decision left only the much less popular saline implants available to patients not involved in clinical research projects.

Plastic surgeons were fearful that saline implants also might be taken off the market.

The ASPRS's immediate reaction was an aggressive media campaign to condemn the FDA-imposed moratorium. At one point the society publicly asked for someone in the Bush administration to overrule the FDA decision. It also sent letters to fifty thousand surgeons in other specialties to warn that other medical products were likely to come under FDA scrutiny. The focus of ASPRS efforts, however, began to change after its own Silicone Implant Research Committee reviewed the ninety key documents that caused the FDA ruling and concluded that these documents did not provide evidence of implant safety. Instead, they raised questions about the manufacturers' business practices. In the year after the FDA decision, the position of the ASPRS evolved gradually from FDA adversary to FDA partner and women's health advocate. The society did the following:

- Responded aggressively to media stories claiming plastic surgeons ignored women's safety;
- Asked members to emphasize the "caring side" of the specialty to reporters;
- Called for research proposals to be reviewed by the Plastic Surgery Educational Foundation for funding;
- Asked to be included in a task force to prioritize research funded by the U.S. Department of Health and Human Services;
- Met with insurance company executives to urge continued coverage of breast reconstruction after mastectomy;
- Established a Breast Implant Patient Relations Network to provide worried women free telephone consultations and a visit if necessary to advise them that the risks of removal might outweigh the risk of the devices.

The society also sent representatives to infiltrate breast-implant consumer groups, such as the Command Trust Network, to understand the issues that caused these women to organize (*Plastic Surgery News* 1993a). The representatives estimated that these groups represent about twenty thousand women whose main goal was obtaining money from manufacturers and, to a lesser degree, plastic surgeons. They reported that some of the speakers also questioned ASPRS public relations efforts to develop articles about cosmetic surgery in magazines and the financing program. Reaching out to these women to establish a more positive relationship was, as one ASPRS leader put it, among the final tasks of the breast implant campaign. It is also part of the larger task to repair the public image of the specialty.

Reconstructing the Public Image

The breast implant crisis took the ASPRS and other physicians involved with breast implants by surprise. The ASPRS had worked closely with implant manufacturers. Surgitek, the manufacturer of polyurethane foam-coated silicone-gel implants, was given the society's first "President's Award" for cosponsoring the 1988 video tele conferences (*Plastic Surgery News* 1988c). Dow Corning had been a longtime, trusted supplier of medical devices for plastic surgery. The company assured the ASPRS that it would have no trouble obtaining FDA approval and did not reveal that it was involved in mounting litigation over the safety of its implants (Hait 1994, 92A–98A). By fall of 1993 more than ten thousand federal and state lawsuits had been filed, involving an estimated fifteen hundred to two thousand plastic surgeons. The 1993–1994 president of the ASPRS summed up the feelings of many plastic surgeons, "I could not have imaged the breast implant decision would turn out as it did. We have a tendency to feel that because we were right, we would win. We were played for fools by manufacturers" (Hait 1994, 98A).

Other plastic surgeons pointed a finger of blame at pressures from the religious right and the politically correct left, pressures which were exerted on the FDA through Congress (Hait 1994, 93A). They felt victimized by the 1990 congressional hearings held by a self-appointed FDA "watch-dog" who filled the congressional record with horror stories of breast implant complications (95A). Still others believed that the Trial Lawyers Association somehow orchestrated the crisis for its members' financial gain (98A). All felt they were under attack by the media, which suddenly filled with stories of betrayal by physicians and the FDA. Reporter Connie Chung was singled out as the plastic surgeons' prime enemy. Her December 1990 "Face-to-Face" broadcast provided the first strongly negative national coverage of breast implants. After the show aired ASPRS members experienced a sharp decrease in the number of patients seeking implants (*Plastic Surgery News* 1992a, 10). The ASPRS was incensed when CBS decided to rebroadcast the show four days before the 1991 FDA hearing to decide the fate of implants and would not include interviews with plastic surgeons or air a thirty-second paid advertisement advising women to phone the society for more information on breast implants.

Many in the media viewed the ASPRS campaign to influence the FDA's decision as financially motivated and self-serving. This view resulted in a temporary, but strong, backlash against physician authority over cosmetic surgery. The media attack was, according to a *New York Times* reporter, triggered by "the scent of deceit" emitted from the conflict between plastic surgeons and the FDA (Larson et al. 1994, 323). A narrative analysis of breast implant articles in newspapers and popular magazines at the peak of the crisis in 1991 and 1992 reveals that the majority included examples of women who had a "horror story" to tell and depicted plastic surgeons as the uncaring "antagonists" who often misled women about the risks or who were inept surgeons (Vanderford et al. 1995). Plastic surgeons also were depicted as "combatants" with other physicians and the FDA, who dared to raise questions about the health risks of implants; and plastic surgeons were portrayed as "profit-oriented business persons" rather than altruistic healers. Some articles reminded readers that plastic surgeons had recommended other procedures, such as painful closed capsulotomies, to break up hardened scar tissue around implants, which increased ruptures and, consequently, health risks. The implication of these depictions was that plastic surgeons could not be trusted. The media had escaped the ASPRS "harness" and were running amok.

The media are important sources of health information, particularly when they saturate the public with reports of a "crisis." A 1991–1992 study of women who had breast implants reports that more than 90 percent cited television as a major source of their information about implants (Palcheff-Wiemer et al. 1993). Women's magazines and newspapers also are mentioned by a majority, although they reportedly have less impact because they lack the more intense visual dimension of television. Before the FDA moratorium 39 percent of those whose breasts were augmented acknowledged feeling differently about their implants after exposure to the media coverage. After the moratorium, during the peak of media coverage, 61 percent said that the media changed their feelings about breast implants. Few breast-reconstructed women reported being influenced by the media in the first survey; however, 59 percent felt differently in the second survey. Satisfaction with their decision to have breast implants declined from 98 percent of all women in the sample to 75 percent.

To assess the damage to the public image of plastic surgeons in 1992, the ASPRS conducted a telephone survey of five hundred women immediately after the moratorium (Palcheff-Wiemer et al. 1993). Only

64 percent described plastic surgeons as somewhat or very believable about breast implants. The society also sponsored focus-group discussions with women thirty-five to fifty-five years old in three major cities and interviewed journalists, editors of women's magazines, and producers of daytime talk shows. Members learned that "The bad news is that the unflattering—and usually inaccurate—stereotype of the arrogant, money-grubbing cosmetic surgeon is still alive and well" (*Plastic Surgery News* 1992b, 1). The only good news was that reconstructive surgery is still universally regarded as important. Even the good news was not that good because the women did not recognize that reconstructive work is done by plastic surgeons. Instead, women associated plastic surgeons only with cosmetic surgery.

The society retrenched to its respected reconstructive roots. Members were advised to emphasize their reconstructive training, experience, and services. The society began to debate changing its name to the American Society for Plastic Surgery. Supporters argued that including reconstructive in the name would lead people to think that the society contains two different types of physicians—reconstructive and plastic surgeons. The latter they associate only with cosmetic surgery. Supporters argued that the name change was necessary to emphasize to the public that physicians who do cosmetic surgery are the same as those who do reconstructive. Opponents, in contrast, feared that deleting reconstructive from their name would define them all in the public's mind as only cosmetic surgeons. After seven years of debate, the name was changed to the American Society of Plastic Surgeons in 1999.

The degree of the rebound to reconstructive legitimacy was evident in the selection of the 1992–1993 ASPRS president, Elvin Zook, an academic whose work is primarily reconstructive and whose views on cosmetic surgery are radical. He advised his colleagues: "More than 10 years ago I was asked what plastic surgery should do to remain viable for the next 50 years. My answer was to give cosmetic surgery to someone else. Cosmetic surgery is the most dangerous surgery. People think all we do is cosmetic surgery, that we're a bunch of hairdressers. That is a danger. Our public image must be that of serious surgeons" (Hait 1994, 88A).

Although his view undoubtedly resonates with some of the plastic surgeons who have complained in editorials and letters to the editor over the last three decades about the increasing prevalence of cosmetic surgery, few rank-and-file plastic surgeons would be willing to give up what has become a large portion of their practice in such a competitive time. There has been, nevertheless, a discernible shift in the public presentation of the specialty to emphasize reconstructive work, altruistic activities, and scientific research on outcomes and to de-emphasize conflict with other specialties and the FDA.

The large amount of media attention given to a classic triumph-over-tragedy story in the wake of the breast implant crisis reinforced the value of the specialty's reconstructive work for its public image. A young man had both of his arms severed when he fell into farm equipment. Although alone, he managed under the traumatic circumstances to return home and call for help. Because of his initiative, relatively little time elapsed and plastic surgeons were able to reattach his arms. His stoic courage and the dramatic nature of the reconstructive surgery engaged the media for weeks, generating highly favorable, image-enhancing coverage for plastic surgeons. In response, the ASPRS reminded members to call their newspapers and contact the society's Communications Department if they were involved in any dramatic reconstructive work. Two of three ASPRS-sponsored Public Education Awards for Excellence in Plastic Surgery Journalism that same year were given to media coverage of complex reconstructive work. The video news release from the annual ASPRS meeting similarly featured dramatic before and after "morphing" of patients, most of whom had reconstructive surgery.

Improving the image of plastic surgeons was the number one ASPRS priority in 1994 (*Plastic Surgery News* 1993d). The ASPRS sought more media coverage of members who participated in volunteer programs. The association began to provide regular coverage of members' volunteer activities in *Plastic Surgery News* and to issue press releases. Most examples involved reconstructive surgery programs in Third World countries, although some were about surgeons who donated their time to local victims of domestic violence and to the removal of gang tattoos. The ASPRS also initiated several domestic public service campaigns in 1994 (*Plastic Surgery News* 1995c). The first was a joint effort with the AMA, the American Academy of Pediatricians, and the American Academy of Dermatology to educate the public about the health hazards of the summer sun. A second sought to educate families about the dangers of firecrackers. The third, cosponsored with Neutrogena Corporation, focused on breast-reconstruction options, how to respond to accidental digit amputation, and how to reduce children's risk of household burns. For the most part, these announcements appeared in women's magazines.

The incoming 1996 president of the ASPRS likened the society to a phoenix that had to reinvent itself after the breast implant crisis (Brody 1996b). It did this by abandoning its adversarial relationship with the FDA and adopting a new partnership based on a renewed commitment to scientific research, the commitment that underpins the legitimacy of modern medical authority. Members now help to recruit patients for manufacturers' clinical studies of cosmetic and reconstructive devices and contribute to the databases needed for long-term follow-up studies. They also have established the National Endowment for Plastic Surgery to raise five million dollars for research by 2000 (*Plastic Surgery News* 1996b). This endowment has focused on outcome studies of procedures such as breast reduction (*Plastic Surgery News* 1997b).

In 1996 the ASPRS opened an Internet site that provides extensive information on the qualifications of members, procedures, costs, statistics on former patients, appropriate motivations for cosmetic surgery, the need for realistic expectations, and its referral number. The site generated seventy thousand calls for referral in the first year (Iverson 1997). Members can elect to have a homepage set up through the ASPRS site. Many already had individual sites. There is also a media center where the organization posts press releases. Recent releases include statements of the society's support for legislation mandating insurance coverage for treatment of children's appearance deformities and reconstruction after mastectomy. Once again, following the success of the ASPRS website, other physicians' organizations have set up their own sites.

As the media's interest in the breast implant crisis waned, favorable coverage of new trends in cosmetic surgery resumed. Talk show hosts, reporters, and journalists focused on aging baby boomers, male cosmetic surgery, fat lips, lasers, endoscopic facelifts, and new liposuction techniques. A popular television series, *Chicago Hope*, featured a plastic surgeon as a sympathetic central character who does more than just cosmetic surgery. The ASPRS assisted in developing the character's role by supplying videos of procedures. It was not long before the editors at *Marie Claire* and other magazines reverted to articles such as "Knifestyles of the Rich and Famous" and Phil Donahue hosted a beauty pageant of former cosmetic surgery patients with an award for the "most improved." The former leader of the breast implant expose, Connie Chung, turned her attention to the "performance art" of a woman who had seven of twenty planned surgeries to give her the eyes of Diana, lips of Europa, nose of Psyche, forehead of Mona Lisa, and chin of Venus. Although the ASPRS wants more attention paid to the reconstructive work of plastic surgeons, the media and the public remain more interested in sensational stories, whether about reconstructive or cosmetic patients or cutting-edge procedures.

Internal Public Relations

The issue of the image of plastic surgeons within medicine was raised in the mid-1970s by ASPRS president Rex Peterson (Hait 1994, 72A). This concern was overtaken by concern about the FTC's imposed deregulation of advertising and subsequent antitrust complaint against the ASPRS's use of board certification as a gatekeeping criteria. The issue of image was raised again at the 1986 ASPRS marketing conference. Although the conference's focus was the specialty's external image, participants were well aware that the expanded plastic work of otolaryngologists, ophthalmologists, and dermatologists threatened plastic surgeons' claims to special expertise and reduced referrals for both reconstructive and cosmetic work from other physicians (*Plastic Surgery News* 1986c). Moreover, turf battles in the 1970s and 1980s with other specialties doing plastic work, particularly in cosmetic surgery and hand surgery, had engendered their animosity. Some other physicians who observed plastic surgeons' sometimes vicious verbal assaults on competitors condemned their unwillingness to compromise for the good of the medical profession. Studies also reveal that plastic surgeons were less available to accept emergency room cases than all but neurosurgeons (Zook 1993). Their absence not only gave reconstructive cases to otolaryngologists and oral surgeons by default, but also damaged plastic surgeons' image within medicine. Leaders in the 1990s repeatedly urged members to "get back into the action" and become involved in hospitals and county medical associations.

Efforts to enhance the image of plastic surgeons within the medical community were overtaken again, this time by the breast implant crisis. By 1993 the crisis abated and the ASPRS turned its attention once again to restoring the public image of the specialty and its internal image and position within medicine. That year the society not only mailed *Procedures in Plastic Surgery* and *Plastic Surgeons: A Delin-*

eation of Qualifications for Clinical Privileges to twenty-five hundred managed care administrators and key hospital administrators, but also sent the former to thirty thousand primary care physicians (*Plastic Surgery News* 1995c). The society produced slide presentations on pediatric plastic surgery, breast reconstruction, hand surgery, and wound care for members to show to colleagues in other specialties. The society set up exhibits at the scientific meetings of other specialties, including the American Academy of Pediatrics, the American Academy of Family Physicians, the American College of Emergency Physicians, and the American College of Obstetricians and Gynecologists, to explain about the special expertise that board-certified plastic surgeons offer their patients. Finally, the society actively sought to defuse the interspecialty battle over cosmetic surgery, the subject of the next chapter. This battle had not been good for business.

5 Sibling Rivalry

The Intraprofessional "Turf War" over Cosmetic Surgery

The blanket nature of a medical license and the breakdown of informal controls over the practice of medicine facilitated the growth of cosmetic surgery. They also resulted in a turf war among the physicians attracted to the surgical challenge, freedom from third-party payers, and financial reward of this work. Territorial claims have a long history in plastic surgery despite its interdisciplinary origin, discussed in chapter 3. These territorial assertions of dominion have been both literal claims to regions of the country and metaphorical claims to surgical procedures. Some of the early leaders, for example, required student apprentices to sign statements that they would not practice within a hundred or more miles (Hait 1994, 51A). The rapid growth in the number of plastic surgeons following World War II ultimately doomed these geographic "fiefdoms." It also doomed the secrecy that surrounded cosmetic operations until the late 1960s.

Although plastic surgeons have been involved in work disputes with orthopedic hand surgeons, oral surgeons, general surgeons, and others, this chapter focuses on the larger, bloodier battle over cosmetic surgery. It begins with some background on the events that led to the hostilities within the brotherhood of physicians. Next, follows a review of plastic surgeons' major "campaigns" to control their rivals through restrictions on medical advertising, specialty licensure, and accreditation of ambulatory surgery sites. These efforts culminated in the 1989 congressional hearings, *Unqualified Doctors Performing Cosmetic Surgery,* from which none of the specialties involved with cosmetic surgery emerged unscathed (U.S. House 1989a,b,c). Since then, these specialties have made some efforts toward detente, although plastic surgeons have yet to cede any occupational ground in a formal treaty. The chapter concludes with a discussion of the potential for turf battles to undermine the professional authority of physicians.

Issues of Dispute

After the American Board of Plastic Surgery was founded in 1937 and given membership in the American Board of Medical Specialties (ABMS) in 1941, training in plastic surgery evolved from preceptorships to comprehensive residency programs including clinical and laboratory work. Admission to these programs required first two, then three years of general surgery experience. This policy changed in the 1950s when Reed Dingman, chair of the American Board of Plastic Surgery, opened his plastic surgery residencies to surgeons with other types of prior training, including otolaryngologists and orthopedic surgeons (Hait 1994, 52A). His actions dismayed many, if not most, of his plastic surgeon colleagues. They argued that sharing techniques would create interspecialty competition for patients, foreshadowing events to come. For the most part, otolaryngologists and other specialists had been shut out of formal training in plastic surgery after World War I. Yet a few had pursued informal training aggressively, especially for nasal work, and founded the American Academy of Facial Plastic and Reconstructive Surgery in 1964.

As early as 1957 the president of the American Society of Plastic and Reconstructive Surgeons (ASPRS) warned members that "intensive rivalry between our specialty and other groups . . . is a direct challenge to our survival. . . . we must accept this challenge and combat it through all the means at our disposal" (Williams et al. 1978, 17). One means has been to distribute materials to members to heighten concern about the incursion of other specialties into the "domain" of plastic surgeons. Another has been to promote publicity that establishes plastic surgeons as the sole authorities in reconstructive and cosmetic surgery.

Public Disparagement

The first interspecialty conflict occurred when Jack Anderson, a resident in otolaryngology, was assigned to the surgical service of a plastic surgeon who refused to allow him into the operating room and hung a towel over the window to prevent him from observing procedures (Hait 1994, 53A). The effort to exclude, rather than incorporate, this otolaryngologist appears in hindsight to have been an inflammatory strategy. This same otolaryngologist subsequently recruited others and led them into battle against plastic surgeons in the "war of the magazines" (Hait 1994, 56A–58A). The first skirmish erupted when *Harper's Bazaar* published an article on "cosmetic plastic surgery" in 1960. The few previous articles on plastic surgery—mostly about reconstructive procedures—had appeared in newspapers and magazines such as *Good Housekeeping. Cosmopolitan, Look, Saturday Evening Post*, and *Newsweek*. Most were a result of the initial public relations efforts of the ASPRS in the 1950s. Unlike previous articles, however, the *Harper's Bazaar* article warned readers contemplating cosmetic surgery to contact the American Board of Plastic Surgery to ensure that their physician was competent: "Some ear, nose and throat men (otolaryngologists) feel qualified to perform the nasal plastics—essentially an elementary cosmetic operation—and no law can stop them. For your own protection, since your aim is maximum aesthetic results, be sure that your surgeon has the added years of study and experience which the American Board of Plastic Surgery certification guarantees" (Trotta 1960, 126).

This public attack on the credibility and competence of other physicians violated a fundamental medical taboo in 1960. Physicians had worked hard to set aside their differences in order to consolidate their authority and achieve cultural legitimacy and respect in the first half of the twentieth century. Although the statement was written by a journalist, in the context of the article it appeared to be the view of plastic surgeons. The reemergence of one group of physicians appearing to question the competence of another in a public forum threatened the cohesiveness of the profession. The reaction was swift and vehement. The otolaryngologists' society sent reprints of the article challenging their competence to every otolaryngologist in the United States and Canada. The recipients, in turn, sent letters to protest the "blatant commercialism" of plastic surgeons and their specialty organization, the ASPRS, both to the American Board of Plastic Surgery and to the Advisory Board of Medical Specialties, the predecessor to the American Board of Medical Specialties. Jack Anderson personally presented his complaint against plastic surgeons to the American Academy of Ophthalmology and Otolaryngology and to the Advisory Board of Medical Specialties. For the first time the organization supported the self-designated "facial plastic and reconstructive" specialists among its members. Another otolaryngologist sent copies of the article with an accompanying letter to the Judicial Council of the American Medical Association (AMA) and to ten thousand organizations and physicians in the United States and Canada to demand the resignation of every ASPRS member, virtually all of the country's board-certified plastic surgeons, from the AMA.

The AMA did not banish ASPRS members. However, the prestigious Advisory Board of Medical Specialties reprimanded the American Board of Plastic Surgery. It also recommended that the ASPRS inform every magazine and newspaper publisher in the country that they may not use the name of the American Board of Plastic Surgery in any articles they print. In accordance with the multi-specialty organization's policy, such a ban would preclude reporters and journalists from using board certification as evidence of the superior expertise of one group of physicians over another equally qualified group. Instead of retreating apologetically and following the directive, the American Board of Plastic Surgery fired back by distributing a *Mademoiselle* article that advised readers to choose a surgeon qualified by the American Board of Otolaryngology for cosmetic rhinoplasty work. The first line in the battle over cosmetic surgery was drawn between these two specialties in the pages of women's magazines.

A 1961 pamphlet distributed by the ASPRS to the public acknowledged that some other specialists offer plastic surgery procedures. However, it labeled them "so-called specialists" without "the respect of medical colleagues [or] the confidence of most patients." The society also worked with the popular press, continuing to urge reporters and journalists to tell readers to seek board-certified plastic surgeons. This remains the central theme in information disseminated by the society, as discussed in the previous chapter. Since 1976 the society has published the booklet "How to Select a Surgeon" for the press and public (Hait 1994, 71A). Plastic surgeons' concern about other specialties encroaching on their medical domain increased along with the demand for cosmetic surgery. A 1971 study confirmed their fears; more than half of the physicians who publicly designated themselves as plastic surgeons at that time were not certified by the American Board of Plastic Surgery (Hait 1994, 69A).

The executive director of the ASPRS prepared a memorandum in 1973 that outlined a "Cold War" to freeze the competition using "guerrilla" tactics while wearing a "political mask of constant negotiation" as a "stalling technique" (U.S. House 1989a, 91–92). Otolaryngologists asserted that the guerrilla tactics included developing and financing a "patently groundless malpractice action" against the plastic surgeons' old foe, Jack Anderson, who by then was a full professor on the faculties of two medical schools and the author of two textbooks and more than eighty scientific articles. One of Anderson's former patients testified in a malpractice case that plastic surgeons urged him to bring the suit and promised to pay his legal fees if he would help them drive out the "quacks" from Anderson's "school" who were "trained in their garages" (U.S. House 1989a, 385–389). The jury found Anderson innocent of malpractice.

In 1975 the executive director of the ASPRS prepared another memorandum on a strategy for dealing with the competitive threat from other specialties. This document noted that the plastic surgeons "have the power, ability and cohesiveness of our members to stall and frustrate the majority of efforts [by competitors] to achieve national recognition from organized medical societies" (qtd. in U.S. House 1989a, 387). That same year, the state medical journal in Arizona published an attack on otolaryngologists authored by local physicians, "Things Are Never What They Seem, Skim Milk Masquerades as Cream" (Crane 1983, 26). The article appeared again in 1982 in the Georgia state medical journal. This time it was published under the name of a physician who would later assume the presidency of ASPRS in 1985. A section added to the article attacked Anderson by name, accusing him of being a quack who formed the American Academy of Facial Plastic and Reconstructive Surgery and American Board of Cosmetic Surgery as a "smoke screen" to hide his lack of qualifications. Anderson and the American Academy of Facial Plastic and Reconstructive Surgery, which is recognized by the AMA and the American College of Surgeons although not by the American Board of Medical Specialties, filed a defamation suit and won a $1.5 million judgment. Anderson donated his settlement to the Education and Research Foundation of the American Academy of Facial Plastic and Reconstructive Surgery (Simons and Hill 1989). In spite of these two defeats for plastic surgeons, the battle over who is competent to perform cosmetic surgery continues on other fronts. The issue of hospital privileges has been particularly contentious.

Hospital Privileges

Otolaryngologists and other specialists who use some plastic procedures complain that they are denied hospital privileges for procedures within their anatomical area of expertise by plastic surgeons' hegemony (Williams et al. 1978, 23–33). The issue of competition between specialties and the increasing difficulty of obtaining hospital privileges to do procedures involving plastic techniques was discussed at the 1969 meeting of the otolaryngologists' American Academy of Facial Plastic and Reconstructive Surgery. A meeting between this group and the ASPRS failed to resolve the problem. Jack Anderson, on behalf of the facial academy, then sent a letter to hospital administrators and executive directors of medical societies in 1971 explaining the potential for abuse if they relied only on certification by the American Board of Plastic Surgery to grant hospital privileges for plastic procedures. Subsequently, when hospitals inquired about certification criteria and the scope of the specialty's practice, the American Board of Otolaryngology sent a packet of material. The packet contained a letter explaining that board-certified otolaryngologists are trained in plastic procedures of the head and neck, an information pamphlet that says members of the specialty are trained in plastic surgery, and a list of procedures which includes some of the same ones on a list of plastic surgery procedures previously sent by the ASPRS to hospitals.

Trying to stop what they perceived as an escalating threat to their specialty, the American Board of Plastic Surgery complained to the American Board of Medical Specialties about these documents. The multi-specialty organization, which includes the American Board of Otolaryngology, determined that the American Board of Otolaryngology's statements were accurate. Failing to enlist the support of other specialty boards in its quest for monopolistic rights to plastic procedures, plastic surgeons were forced to negotiate with otolaryngologists. After several years of discussion, both boards issued a joint statement in 1974 that acknowledged the two specialties have some overlapping interests and experience and urged hospital administrators, medical schools, credential committees, and local medical societies to determine physicians' qualifications and issue privileges on an individual basis. The latter part of this statement concerning determination of qualifications merely reiterated the explicit polices of both the American Board of Medical Specialties and the AMA. Both continue to maintain that physicians should be judged on broad indicators of their individual competence, not merely board certification.

The American Board of Otolaryngology signed the joint statement in good faith and assumed that the attacks on their qualifications to do plastic surgery in the head and neck region in hospitals would cease (Williams et al. 1978, 27–33). Instead, the American Board of Plastic Surgery repudiated the joint statement in letters to approximately fifty ASPRS members. In these letters, the board indicated that its certification was the only "ticket" to the practice of plastic surgery. When otolaryngologists sought to update their Essentials for Approved Residency Programs in Otolaryngology to include the plastic and reconstructive procedures of the head and neck, procedures that were already being taught in their programs, the ASPRS fought to have the American College of Surgeons veto the change. The plastic surgeons' organization, however, was unsuccessful and the change went into effect in 1975.

The Federal Trade Commission (FTC) initiated a two-year antitrust investigation of the ASPRS in 1976 and subpoenaed all of its records. When the society's Chicago attorneys recommended compliance, the president hired a more aggressive Washington firm with FTC experience. Following this firm's advice, the society only handed over some documents to answer the complaint and began to negotiate (Hait 1994, 72A). This response echoed the cold war strategy of constant negotiation and stalling used by the ASPRS with its sibling rivals. The FTC's 1978 memorandum recommended that an official complaint be filed against the society. It also noted the incomplete nature of the submitted material and the need for additional "post complaint discovery" (Williams et al. 1978, 8–9). In spite of attempts to censor the documents given to the FTC, the investigation revealed abundant evidence of a turf war.

The FTC documented local plastic surgeons' actions to block other specialists, mainly otolaryngologists, from gaining hospital privileges for plastic surgery operations in areas of anatomical expertise in seventeen states (Williams et al. 1978, 27–33). Even when otolaryngologists had hospital privileges for some regional plastic procedures, there were sometimes problems. Some had their hospital privileges challenged by plastic surgeons and, in a few cases, revoked by hospitals. Others encountered overt personal hostility from plastic surgeons. In an extreme case, a Colorado plastic surgeon physically barred an otolaryngologist from entering an operating room where his patient was waiting for a facelift.

The FTC investigation provided evidence of duplicity in plastic surgeons' claims that they only seek to protect the public from harm when they oppose granting hospital privileges to other specialists for plastic procedures in regional areas of anatomical expertise. Transcripts from meetings of the governing body of the American Board of Plastic Surgery recorded the specialty's leaders' statements:

> I think that nobody at this table would deny that there are good ENTs [the acronym for ear, nose, and throat specialists, an alternative name for otolaryngologists] and ophthalmologists who do cosmetic and plastic and facial and head and neck surgery. . . .
>
> I do not think it is very hard to learn to do aesthetic surgery and I think that is why ENT, among other reasons, has gone for it. . . .
>
> I think it is probably true, if you place a generalist against a regionalist, the regionalist is going to win most of the time. (qtd. in Williams et al. 1978, 22)

This duplicity led the FTC to submit a proposed complaint and relief order to the ASPRS in 1978 for restraining the trade of other physicians equally qualified to do some types of plastic surgery. The FTC's proposed complaint charged that the ASPRS's anticompetitive practices included not only disparaging the competence, ability, and training of others and preventing them from obtaining hospital privileges, but also refusing to publish advertisements for meetings of their organizations, trying to prevent the instruction in plastic surgery techniques to nonplastic surgeons, and restricting inclusion in directory listings of plastic surgeons. The ASPRS argued that the real issue that should be under FTC scrutiny was the "deceptive" advertising of cosmetic surgery by nonplastic surgeon competitors.

Refusing Advertisements
and Announcements

Plastic and Reconstructive Surgery, the official journal of the ASPRS, is widely read by physicians who do plastic procedures, including non-ASPRS members. Consequently, it is the most visible forum for disseminating information about plastic surgery. The journal contains articles about clinical practice and research, editorials, announcements about symposia and continuing education programs, and advertisements about new medical devices and pharmaceutical products. Since the 1970s, the journal has included extensive coverage of cosmetic surgery in addition to reconstructive surgery.

Despite its broad audience, the FTC charged that the journal had a de facto policy to reject papers and advertisements for continuing education programs and symposia submitted by nonplastic surgeons until 1975 (Williams et al. 1978, 33–37). At that time, the Board of Plastic Surgery was lobbying against revisions in the Essentials for Approved Residency Programs in Otolaryngology. These essentials define the scope of practice for otolaryngologists and are used by hospitals and others to determine qualifications. On the advice of counsel and consistent with the cold war strategy, the Executive Committee of the ASPRS passed a resolution stating, "in no way do we wish to restrain anyone's trade." The committee then rejected the facial academy's advertisement for publication in the journal. Instead, the ASPRS published the announcement as a small classified advertisement in *Plastic Surgery News*. the ASPRS newsletter sent to members. A letter to the advertising editor of the journal from the ASPRS explained the contradictory actions of the Executive Committee. It stated, "The previously established philosophy of not accepting the Facial Academy's advertising in the journal was reaffirmed. It would be best not to respond to Dr. Tandy or any similar individuals who request space . . . so that there can't possibly be any legal repercussions." The FTC claimed in 1978 that only a token few nonplastic surgeon publication requests were granted up to that time, in spite of the society's assertion that its publications were open to all.

Restricting Access to Instruction in Plastic Techniques

Post-residency training is vital for physicians. Both the AMA and the American Board of Medical Specialties maintain that residency training alone does not qualify a physician to perform all procedures in a specialty. Moreover, medical knowledge constantly expands. With this expansion come innovations in surgical techniques and medical technology. To stay up-to-date, physicians must participate in continuing education. A central function of specialty organizations is to promote opportunities for post-residency training. These programs can range from short, specialized workshops to longer, more formal training programs like fellowships under other physicians.

The FTC charged that the ASPRS denied other physicians access to programs sponsored by plastic surgeons and pressured individual plastic surgeons to avoid instructing other physicians (Williams 1978, 37–41). Both the ASPRS and its allied organization, the American Society for Aesthetic Plastic Surgeons, closed their scientific and educational meetings to nonmembers until 1972. At that time the ASPRS officially opened its educational meetings to protect the tax-exempt status of its Educational Foundation. Nevertheless, the FTC claimed that its closed-door policy continued informally because the organization limits registration and members learn about meetings before nonmembers.

The FTC also provided evidence that the ASPRS discouraged plastic surgeons from participating in the programs of rival specialties. The November 1972 newsletter published a statement from the Inter–professional Relations Committee that said, "[P]articipation by members of our society in commercially-sponsored, recreation-oriented meetings purporting to teach principles and techniques of plastic surgery (Fourth International Congress of Ophthalmic Surgery, International Academy of Cosmetic Surgery, etc.) should be censured" (Williams 1978, 37–41). At the time of this statement little training in cosmetic surgery was available in plastic surgeons' residency programs. Physicians who wanted to do cosmetic work had to look for training wherever they could find it. Numerous plastic surgeons were chastised or ostracized by colleagues for participating in multi-specialty programs in cosmetic surgery. For example, an associate clinical professor of plastic surgery at the University of Colorado was threatened with termination if he participated in the 1976 Vail Cosmetic Surgery Program. He withdrew. The Interprofessional Relations Committee published a second resolution in 1977 stating that members should cease conducting short courses for nonplastic surgeons, appearing on panels and teaching seminars with nonplastic surgeons, and publishing articles in nonplastic surgeon journals.

The wrangling over liposuction shows the degree of importance physicians attach to post-residency training as a basis for claiming occupational rights to new medical technology. In the 1970s some European surgeons began to experiment with reducing fat accumulations using a suction tube. Pierre Fournier, a French plastic surgeon who had studied with the pioneers of liposuction, Giorgio Fischer of Rome and Yves-Gerard Illouz of Paris, introduced the procedure at the 1980 meeting of the American Society for Dermatologic Surgery (American Society for Dermatologic Surgery 1989). Otolaryngologists, general surgeons, plastic surgeons, dermatologists, and others involved in founding the American Board of Cosmetic Surgery invited Fournier to talk about the procedure at their January 1982 meeting (Newman 1989). Gregory Hetter, board certified in both plastic surgery and otolaryngology, attended this presentation. Convinced of liposuction's enormous cosmetic potential, he and four other plastic surgeons went to Paris six months later to watch Illouz operate. The race to claim territorial rights to a technique the media later referred to as "every woman's dream come true" was underway.

The Europeans were invited to discuss their work at the 1982 annual ASPRS meeting held in the fall (Hait 1994, 79A). Their presentation attracted considerable attention. The cosmetic surgeons' group held their first live operating room workshop about the same time and incorporated a new specialty association, the American Society of Liposuction Surgery, in December (Newman 1989). When Hetter invited Illouz to teach a short course for plastic surgeons, he discovered Illouz had already agreed to teach a course for the cosmetic surgeons' group in February 1983 (Hait 1994, 79A). Fearing that plastic surgeons had been outflanked by the multi-specialty cosmetic surgeons' group, Hetter formed a legal partnership with Illouz and Fournier, Lipolysis, Inc., which preempted the French surgeons from teaching for the cosmetic surgeons' association. Hetter then began to organize a symposium for American plastic surgeons.

The ASPRS leadership was distressed that Hetter had acted on his own and requested that he turn Lipolysis over to the Educational Foundation, which is controlled by the ASPRS (Hait 1994, 79A–80A). When he only agreed to turn over the symposium he was planning, Hetter found himself cast aside. He was not appointed to the plastic surgeons' committee to investigate Illouz's technique, and more powerful ASPRS members took over the symposium. As a result, Hetter started his own professional organization, the Lipolysis Society, and scheduled its first scientific meeting to coincide with the next ASPRS meeting in the fall of 1983. The Lipolysis Society's name was changed to Lipoplasty Society of North America, a name undoubtedly chosen to associate the technique with plastic surgery. According to Hait's (1994) official history of the ASPRS, this organization has not been integrated fully with other mainstream plastic surgery organizations, as have previous "renegade" groups like the American Society for Aesthetic Plastic Surgeons and even the ASPRS itself. A decade later, the former ASPRS president in charge of the liposuction investigation still objected to Hetter's contention that he had loaded the study committee with fellow members of the American Society of Aesthetic Plastic Surgery. In a letter to the editor about the official ASPRS history he claimed that Hetter was "jaded and prejudiced" and suggested it was time "to extinguish the smoldering embers of personal vendettas and/or any residual intersocietal hostility" (Fredricks 1995). A response to his letter points out that his remark "only serves to open old wounds" (Burnham 1996).

The wounds created by liposuction are deep between specialties as well. All physicians involved with cosmetic surgery immediately realized there was much at stake with liposuction. Within only six years of its introduction in the United States, liposuction became the most frequent cosmetic procedure done by plastic surgeons (American Society of Plastic and Reconstructive Surgeons 1989a) and probably by many other physicians doing cosmetic surgery. The Lipolysis Society responded to prospective patient inquiries with the statement that the "revolutionary plastic surgical technique [was] perfected by Lipolysis-trained, board-certified plastic surgeons" (Newman 1989) at a time when board-certified plastic surgeons were scrambling to take a two- or three-day workshop to learn about the technique, as were other surgeons involved with cosmetic work. The French surgeon Illouz was called a "plastic surgeon" in this same document and in a special April 1989 issue of *Clinics in Plastic Surgery* devoted to liposuction, although Illouz had no formal training in plastic and reconstructive surgery and his practice prior to pioneering liposuction was in abortion and other gynecological procedures. Nevertheless, the special liposuction issue of *Clinics* contained disparaging comments about gynecologists who do liposuction (4), as well as otolaryngologists, general surgeons, and dermatologists (24). The author recommended limiting hospital privileges for the procedure to plastic surgeons.

The introduction to a special October 1988 issue *of Journal of Dermatologic Surgery and Oncology* on liposuction claimed that dermatologists were the innovators and leaders in liposuction. Unlike the plastic surgeons' journal, however, the introduction acknowledged that the procedures are "done competently by otolaryngologists, general surgeons, and general plastic surgeons" (Hanke 1988, 1051). The *Journal of Dermatologic Surgery Oncology* also contained an editorial from French plastic surgeon Fournier, who pointed out that machine-assisted liposuction started a war among surgical specialists in the United States. He further noted that the advent of syringe liposculpturing has broadened its appeal to non-surgeons, while reducing patient risk. He said that he, like the Italian Fischer, whom he called the "father of liposculpturing," believed that "liposculpturing does not belong to a defined surgical specialty. It is a new concept of body contouring using instruments not usually used in normal surgery." He concluded with a warning that physicians need to recognize their own limits because "in all professions it takes ten years to make a reputation for oneself, but less than one minute to lose it" (Fournier 1988, 1055–1056). Since 1976, however, American physicians have found it possible to establish an instant public reputation for cosmetic surgery with a well-financed advertising and public relations campaign.

Deceptive Advertising

Strained relations between plastic surgeons and other physicians involved in cosmetic surgery snapped when the FTC, armed with the 1975 Supreme Court ruling in *Goldfarb v. Virginia State Bar,* forced open the market to medical service advertising. Prior to the extension of antitrust law to the "learned professions," the AMA's code of ethics restricted physicians to advertising only information such as location, hours, and telephone number. More than that, such as descriptions of procedures offered or prices, was considered solicitation and proscribed. As a result of the FTC action, the AMA had to revise its code of ethics to prohibit only false or misleading advertising and to eliminate all distinction between informative advertising and solicitation. The proportion of self-employed physicians who advertise has climbed steadily since then, reaching 32 percent by 1991, up from 10 percent just four years earlier (Kmetik and Emmons 1994, 4). Advertising varies by specialty and is highest, 41 percent, among the surgical subspecialties, whose members spent an average of $4,490 in 1991. Undoubtedly marketing budgets have increased since then.

Plastic surgeons believe their identity and livelihood are jeopardized by the ability of other physicians to advertise themselves as specialists in various types of cosmetic surgery. The leaders of the ASPRS began a vitriolic attack in their journal, *Plastic and Reconstructive Surgery,* and in state medical journals against "the copyists—alien technologies, the self-proclaimed, the untrained, and the unqualified" (Peterson 1978, 490), "the disciplines that claim territorial rights to what we consider to be our property" (Klein 1983, 866). The ASPRS claims that otolaryngologists who call themselves "facial plastic surgeons" and refer to board-certified plastic surgeons as "general plastic surgeons" are trying to mislead the public about who are the "true" specialists (Klein 1983, 866). The ASPRS also complains about those who advertise as "cosmetic surgeons" and "fraudulently" say they are board certified when their board is not one recognized by the American Board of Medical Specialties (Jarrett 1989).

Some of the most bitter controversy centers on physicians who are not board certified in plastic and reconstructive surgery but choose to be included under the specialty in the Yellow Pages (Manstein 1987; Reade and Ratzan 1987). When a county medical society issued a complaint in 1985 to a Texas otolaryngologist who had listed himself under several specialties, including plastic surgery, he reported the incident to the FTC, which ordered the society to stop trying to control nondeceptive advertising (Page 1989a, 50).

The Yellow Pages are an important source of patients. "Physicians and Surgeons" is the most frequently consulted heading in the more than six thousand Yellow Page directories across the country. Survey data indicate that one-third of all adults refer to the Yellow Pages for information about physicians for themselves or other family members (Yellow Pages Publishers Association 1988). Some only look up the telephone number of their regular physician, but 28 percent do not have a specific doctor in mind when they open a directory to look for a physician. The percentage is likely to be higher for those seeking specialized, elective care, such as cosmetic surgery, that would not be covered by managed care insurance companies or would not likely be offered by their family physicians.

Trying to distinguish themselves from competitors in the Yellow Pages, the ASPRS, in conjunction with a national program initiated by the American Board of Medical Specialties, tried placing group listings for members in the Yellow Pages beginning in 1988. The AMA and a number of specialty associations, including otolaryngology and dermatology, opposed the program (*Plastic Surgery News,* 1990a). Local restrictions in many areas also impeded the program and it was terminated (*Plastic Surgery News* 1991a). The ASPRS, nevertheless, continues to encourage members to display their organization's logo in their individual advertisements and to highlight their board certification. The ASPRS further suggests mentioning the requirements for board certification in plastic surgery and the fact that the American Board of Plastic Surgery is "the only ABMS board that is exclusively devoted to plastic surgery and the only ABMS, board that certifies physicians in the full range of plastic and reconstructive procedures" (*Plastic Surgery News* 1994d, 15).

The Campaign for Restrictions on Advertising

The ASPRS does not regard highlighting credentials as sufficient to offset aggressive advertising of cosmetic surgery by other types of physicians in the Yellow Pages and the media. ASPRS leaders have campaigned vigorously for restrictions since advertising was legalized. They have argued that advertisers who claim to be board certified should be required to name their certifying board (Gorney 1989b). This would prevent physicians who advertise cosmetic procedures from implying they are board certified in plastic surgery when their board certification is actually in obstetrics and gynecology, general surgery, or some other specialty. A study commissioned by the ASPRS to demonstrate to the FTC that this type of advertising is deceptive revealed that consumers assume that physicians who advertise cosmetic surgery are board certified in plastic surgery (*Plastic Surgery News,* 1990a). The FTC, nevertheless, declined to require physicians to disclose their certifying board when they identify themselves as board certified.

Plastic surgeons campaigned in California in 1988 for legislation that would have prevented physicians from advertising certification by any board not recognized by the American Board of Medical Specialties (Page 1989a, 49). Under the proposed legislation board-certified otolaryngologists would have been required to list the American Board of Otolaryngology and prevented from listing the American Board of Cosmetic Surgery or the American Board of Facial Plastic and Reconstructive Surgery, even if they also were certified by these boards with more comprehensible names. Otolaryngologists' strong opposition ultimately blocked passage of the bill. They argued that such legislation takes advantage of the general public's lack of familiarity with otolaryngology and, as a result of their "Greek name, incomprehensible to most prospective patients, the general surgeon obtains a strong marketing advantage" (U.S. House 1989a, 90).

Otolaryngologists have long felt handicapped by their obscure name. They previously embraced the informal name ENT, which stands for ear, nose, and throat, the body organs that formed the original basis for the specialty's emergence in the late nineteenth century. When antibiotics and other changes reduced demand for surgical treatment of infection in these organs, otolaryngologists added tumor removal and other surgical interventions to their repertoire and in 1980 appended "Head and Neck Surgery" to the name of the American Academy of Otolaryngology and their journal, the *Archives of Otolaryngology,* to indicate a broader regional area of specialization. Many then began to advertise themselves as head and neck surgeons rather than ENTs. This shift from an organ-based definition of the specialty to a regional one put otolaryngologists at odds with general surgeons. General surgeons argued that there is little basis in physiology to justify a regional specialization and that most surgical specialties—neurosurgery, urology, orthopedics, ophthalmology—are organized according to organ systems and organ functions, as was otolaryngology previously (Friedmann 1989). General surgeons similarly have resisted efforts by others to advertise themselves as abdominal surgeons.

Otolaryngologists involved in facial cosmetic surgery advertise as "facial plastic and reconstructive surgeons," to which plastic surgeons, whom they refer to as "general plastic surgeons," vehemently object. The ASPRS continues to refer to them publicly by their Greek name, "ear, nose, and throat specialists," or even "Brand X" (e.g., Hait 1994, 70A–71A). Otolaryngologists and other types of physicians who advertise as cosmetic surgeons offer the least ambiguity to prospective patients and generate the most hostility from plastic surgeons. Again arguing for truth in advertising, the ASPRS wants the FTC to allow advertising claims of superior qualifications "only if the claims can be substantiated" (American Society of Plastic and Reconstructive Surgeons 1989b, 5). It also wants states to require those who say that they are certified by a board that is not recognized by the American Board of Medical Specialties (ABMS), including the American Board of Cosmetic Surgery and the American Board of Facial and Reconstructive Surgery, to acknowledge the absent recognition. This strategy is designed to deter potential patients who, lacking sufficient knowledge to judge medical competence, rely on institutional endorsements. Plastic surgeons assumed it would also undermine the marketing strategy of some competitors who ambiguously advertise themselves as "ABMS board-certified" members of the American Academy of Cosmetic Surgery or the American Academy of Facial Plastic and Reconstructive Surgery. Because neither of the latter two organizations is a certification board, these physicians could be certified in a board that is recognized by the American Board of Medical Specialties but is not related to any type of surgery, cosmetic or otherwise. Repeated efforts by these organizations to win official recognition of their subspecialty certification by the American Board of Medical Specialties have not yet succeeded.

Despite almost two decades of pressure by board-certified plastic surgeons, the few states that have enacted restrictions on medical advertising have left the door open to determining qualifications. Arizona adopted the first legislation in the 1970s. The statute states that a physician cannot advertise as a specialist "when such is not the case" (Page 1989, 46). The law, however, does not define how to evaluate specialty status. Texas voted in 1988 to require that physicians indicate the full name of the board when they refer to their certified specialty status. Plastic surgeons argue that the Texas law, which reflects the AMA's policy, does not protect consumers who are unlikely to know the difference between a highly regarded specialty board and a "diploma mill." Florida, Oklahoma, and Maryland passed more restrictive regulations in the 1980s favoring the boards recognized by the American Board of Medical Specialties. Each recognizes certification by these boards as indicative of specialty status. The latter two also recognize boards judged by the state medical license board to be equivalent to the boards recognized by the American Board of Medical Specialties. California and Colorado passed similar legislation in 1990 and 1991, respectively (*Plastic Surgery News* 1991c).

In every case, proposals to restrict advertising claims of specialty status have encountered strong opposition from otolaryngologists and other specialists and reticence by the AMA to support such legislation. The AMA argues that physicians should not be too tightly defined by board-certified status because interests often change during careers. Eschewing legal controls, the AMA in 1989 merely urged physicians to state the full names of their certifying boards (Page 1989a, 48). Consequently, the acrimonious fight over advertising medical specialty credentials continues.

The Campaign for Specialty Licensure

Some board-certified plastic surgeons openly advocate establishing a rigid division of labor in medicine with specialty licenses. Although the ASPRS has no official position on specialty licensure, some individual leaders of this organization have called for such a radical restructuring of medical practice. They justify their position in terms of patient safety in light of the increased complexity of medicine: "We're in a high-tech age. It's just not reasonable for physicians with inadequate training to do anything they want" (Page 1989a, 46).

For a brief period during the perceived physician shortage of the

1960s and 1970s, a few states issued specialty licenses. These were given only to physicians, most often in psychiatry, whose training was in question (Page 1989b, 38). All states subsequently discontinued this practice, but two have since revived the policy. Oregon offers limited specialty licenses to physicians licensed in other states who pass an oral exam in their specialty, even though they fail the state's general medical competency test. Massachusetts offers limited licenses to physicians whose medical school's quality is in question. Plastic surgeon advocates of specialty licensure regard these new developments as a first step and claim specialty licensure is necessary and inevitable, now that hospital privileges no longer regulate surgical practices.

Unswayed by such arguments, most organized physician groups, including the AMA, American Board of Medical Specialties, and the Federation of State Medical Boards, oppose specialty licensure. The AMA, for example, uses self-designation to classify medical doctors in its Physician Masterfile, the most comprehensive source of information on medical doctors' training, licensure, board-certification, geographic mobility, and employment. Despite opposition to the idea of specialty licensure by these formal organizations, managed care corporations and hospitals often use board certification as a de facto specialty license requirement when making decisions about hiring and granting hospital privileges. It is also used by insurance providers to determine reimbursement fees. This development is indicative of a natural evolution toward a more rigid division of labor that eventually may culminate in specialty licensure. In the meantime, the ASPRS has adopted the official position that physicians should be allowed to perform cosmetic operations in their offices only if they hold hospital privileges for these same procedures (American Society of Plastic and Reconstructive Surgeons 1989b, 5). They have so far failed to win legislative support for their position.

The American Board of Cosmetic Surgery and the American Board of Facial Plastic and Reconstructive Surgery may finesse the campaign for specialty licensure. They assert that certification in the general field of plastic surgery is too broad to adequately ensure expertise in the rapidly expanding field of cosmetic surgery (U.S. House 1989a, 56–58). In their two- or three-year residency programs, plastic surgeons need to be trained in many specialized areas, including hand surgery, burn surgery, head and neck cancer surgery, maxillofacial surgery, harelip and cleft palate surgery, craniofacial surgery, and trauma surgery, as well as cosmetic surgery. As an alternative to this broad field of training, the American Board of Facial Plastic and Reconstructive Surgery certifies physicians only in head and neck surgery and the American Board of Cosmetic Surgery began to certify physicians in specific regional areas of cosmetic surgery in 1990. However, efforts to gain approval from the American Board of Medical Specialties for official recognition of independent subcertification in regional plastic surgery have met opposition from the American Board of Plastic Surgery.

The Campaign for Accreditation of Ambulatory Surgery Sites

The growth of out-of-hospital surgery has been particularly rapid for cosmetic procedures. As discussed in chapter 4, this trend has contributed to the breakdown of the informal controls over cosmetic surgery previously exerted by plastic surgeons. It has also increased risks. In response, the ASPRS founded the American Association for Accreditation of Ambulatory Plastic Surgery Facilities in 1980 (U.S. House 1989c, 46–55). Accreditation by this association is voluntary and tiered by type of anesthesia used and scope of procedures performed. Facilities must have adequate resuscitation and life-support equipment and emergency procedures in place. Arguing for the need to make such accreditation mandatory, one of the past presidents of this association pointed out, "Even tattoo artists, hairdressers and manicurists need licensing and/or health board examination to practice" (*Plastic Surgery News* 1993c, 12).

The ASPRS choose to establish an independent accreditation organization rather than join the Accreditation Association for Ambulatory Health Care, which grew out of the Joint Commission on Accreditation of Hospitals in 1979. In 1997 this association had accredited about 600 ambulatory care facilities, ranging from office surgery centers and birthing centers to university health services and health maintenance organizations (Accreditation Association for Ambulatory Health Care, 1997, personal communication). ASPRS's professional rivals, the American Academy of Facial Plastic and Reconstructive Surgery and the American Academy of Cosmetic Surgery, are two of the thirteen member organizations of this interdisciplinary association. In contrast, the American Association for Accreditation of Ambulatory Plastic Surgery Facilities only accredits ambulatory surgical facilities owned or directed by board-certified plastic surgeons. Moreover, to be accredited the plastic surgeons have to have malpractice insurance and hospital privileges to perform the same operations at a local hospital.

The impact of voluntary accreditation of ambulatory surgery facilities has been limited. By 1993 only 400 facilities were accredited by the American Association for Accreditation of Ambulatory Plastic Surgery Facilities (*Plastic Surgery News* 1993c). Only one-fourth of practicing plastic surgeons did their cosmetic surgery in such facilities, although the number was increasing. In the mid-1990s the association expanded its oversight to include other surgical specialties, as long as they were recognized by the American Board of Medical Specialties, and dropped "Plastic" from its name (American Association for Accreditation of Ambulatory Surgery Facilities, 1999, personal communications). The vast majority of the 517 facilities accredited by 1997 were staffed by plastic surgeons. An increasing number of newly accredited facilities, however, were staffed by board-certified otolaryngologists, ophthalmologists, obstetricians/gynecologists, and urologists. Some 50 additional facilities were in the process of accreditation review.

Throughout the 1990s the ASPRS, along with several other medical organizations, worked to develop both national and state legislation to make accreditation of office-based, ambulatory surgery facilities mandatory. Success has proved elusive. By 1999, only California had mandatory accreditation legislation in effect. The requirements are not all that the ASPRS wanted. The 1996 California law would not preclude other kinds of physicians from gaining accreditation to do cosmetic surgery in their ambulatory facilities (*Plastic Surgery News* 1996a, 8). Nevertheless, the ASPRS argues that the standards of this association should be mandatory for all sites in which cosmetic surgery takes place.

The 1989 Congressional Hearings on Cosmetic Surgery

Board-certified plastic surgeons moved their campaign to the federal level in the late 1980s. The ASPRS lobbied then Congressman Ron Wyden and other members of the house to shift the focus of the FTC from pursuing professional efforts to constrain advertising to pursuing misleading advertising by competitors (*Plastic Surgery News* 1987c). A subcommittee of the House Committee on Small Business held hearings, *Unqualified Doctors Performing Cosmetic Surgery: Policies and Enforcement: Activities of the Federal Trade*

Commission (U.S. House 1989a,b,c). The hearings initially appeared to be designed to showcase the ASPRS's definition of the cosmetic surgery "problem." Announcing the hearings, the congressional chair, Ron Wyden, said, "Thousands have been disfigured and deformed under the cosmetic surgeon's knife. These terrible consequences show what can happen when any doctor, armed with only a four-year medical degree, can hold himself out as a cosmetic surgeon, or for that matter, as a brain or heart surgeon" (American Society of Plastic and Reconstructive Surgeons 1989b, 2). He opened the hearing with a statement about the "explosive growth" of the "sunrise" cosmetic surgery industry. He condemned the FTC's laissez-faire policy, which he claimed has led to "self-declared medical boards" and "pseudo surgeons" who have "realized huge profits" while causing the "physical and emotional scarring of too many patients" (U.S. House 1989a, 1–2). He deplored the advent of surgery done in physicians' offices away from peer review and normal government monitoring systems. He noted these unregulated office facilities are "touted as institutes, or centers, or clinics of cosmetic surgery in the most expansive ads," even though some "lack the most basic life-support systems" and properly trained assistants. As evidence, he quoted statistics from the ASPRS about eleven deaths from liposuction in the first six and one-half years of this procedure in the United States and referred to deaths, infections, and strokes from other cosmetic procedures.

The chair's opening remarks were followed by two former cosmetic surgery patients who testified to adverse experiences. One stated that her "tummy tuck" at the hands of a cosmetic surgeon resulted in an infection that destroyed her mitral valve. She suffered heart failure five times while other physicians tried to bring her previously unattended infection under control before they could implant an artificial valve. The other testified that she was disabled and deformed by liposuction. Her surgery, however, was performed by a board-certified plastic surgeon.

Referring to these two cases, representatives of the ASPRS next testified that even though bad surgical results occur "even among the most qualified physicians . . . the probability of such an outcome is significantly less when the surgeon . . . is certified by the American Board of Plastic Surgery" (U.S. House 1989a, 19). They did not, however, provide data to support their claims. Instead, they argued for regulation of advertising and out-of-hospital cosmetic surgery and illustrated the potential risks with stories, some accompanied by slides, of disastrous outcomes—ruptured intestines, faces turned into "horror masks," grotesquely deformed noses, a forty-two-year-old woman who cannot stand, sit, or have sexual intercourse after a buttocks lift. Yet, when the chair suggested that cosmetic surgery is "unnecessary" in a question, a plastic surgeon responded that "unnecessary is a very broad term" and deflected the question back to the need for advertising controls because of the risks (31). Anticipating the coming testimony of otolaryngologists and other cosmetic surgeons, this same plastic surgeon said near the end of the session, "I am sure that this afternoon that you will see from the other side all kinds of catastrophes and difficult problems that we have created. It is not exclusive problems. [sic] Everyone has complications. Anyone who does not has a pact with the devil or has not done enough surgery" (36). As a member of a malpractice insurance company's board of directors, this plastic surgeon spoke with expertise about complications.

A past president of both the American Academy of Cosmetic Surgery and the American Academy of Facial Plastic and Reconstructive Surgery, whose unusual background also includes board certification in plastic surgery thirty-five years earlier, also spoke about risks. He testified that board certification in plastic surgery is no guarantee against problems. He claimed that 436 suits were filed in the Los Angeles superior civil court against the 138 active board-certified plastic surgeons in the area between 1979 and the third quarter of 1989 (U.S. House 1989a, 82).

The thrust of the testimony from representatives of both the American Board of Cosmetic Surgery and the American Academy of Facial Plastic and Reconstructive Surgery, however, was not directed at risks. Instead, they focused on the need for consumer choice and a more aggressive FTC to stop the efforts by board-certified plastic surgeons to restrain the trade of other equally, if not better, trained physicians. They gave numerous examples of board-certified plastic surgeons' attempts to block other physicians from doing cosmetic surgery. They argued that plastic surgeons block other physicians from gaining hospital privileges, from attending ASPRS-sponsored continuing education programs, and from advertising in its medical journal. They testified that as a result of the plastic surgeons' political power in medicine, other physicians have a hard time obtaining malpractice insurance to cover cosmetic surgery, *Index Medicus* refuses to list the *Journal of Cosmetic Surgery*. and the AMA refuses to give continuing medical education credits for programs organized by the American Academy of Cosmetic Surgery.

Representatives of both groups asserted, without supplying evidence, that more intensive regional specialization improves cosmetic surgery outcomes. They claimed that their members have a narrow super-specialization that gives them greater expertise than board-certified plastic surgeons. Otolaryngologists from the American Academy of Facial Plastic and Reconstructive Surgery additionally contrasted their more extensive residency and fellowship training in facial surgery with that of "general" plastic surgeons. One mentioned an article, in the ASPRS's journal, that reported approximately half of the graduating plastic surgery residents believe that their training was inadequate (U.S. House 1989a, 93). They also discussed a 1989 ASPRS newsletter article which reported that 63 percent of members think that maintaining a practice in all areas of plastic surgery is impractical. When asked by members of the subcommittee about advertising abuses, they suggested that the biggest abuse is by plastic surgeons who claim to be the best qualified to do plastic surgery. When asked about the difficulty consumers have choosing good physicians, they reiterated the need for consumer choice and otolaryngologists' longer, more specialized training. When asked about risks, they acknowledged that "every surgical procedure has within it an inherent risk and complication" and stressed that patients need to make an informed choice with "complete knowledge of those risks and complications" (105).

The 1989 congressional hearings failed to give board-certified plastic surgeons what they wanted. Their rivals remained free to advertise and continue doing cosmetic surgery in their private offices. Board-certified plastic surgeons lacked the support of the AMA and other specialty associations in their quest for federal regulations. They also lacked statistics to support their claims of superior expertise and outcomes in cosmetic surgery, compared to other physicians. As a result, publicity surrounding the hearings focused more on the turf battle than the health impact of commercial advertising of elective surgery by unregulated practitioners in unregulated private offices. This outcome was unfavorable for plastic surgeons' reputations and economic interests. It also had implications for the reputation of the whole profession and the authority and legitimacy of the American Board of Medical Specialties.

Efforts at Detente

The vocal conflict between plastic surgeons and their sibling rivals, many of whom were certified by other specialty boards in the multidisciplinary American Board of Medical Specialties, threatened the authority of the umbrella organization. Despite the AMA's official position against any rigid division of labor in the medical profession, hospitals and managed care organizations increasingly required board certification by one of the American Board of Medical Specialties member boards as a condition of work. Having physicians certified by different member boards accuse each other of lacking ethics, expertise, and judgement cuts to the heart of the umbrella organization's credibility. It also threatens the unity of the profession.

Both the AMA and the American Board of Medical Specialties continued to pressure board-certified plastic surgeons to compromise with their rivals after the failed attempt at detente in 1974. Two years before the 1989 congressional hearings, the AMA negotiated a joint policy statement on intraprofessional relations between the ASPRS and the American Academy of Otolaryngology—Head and Neck Surgery (*Plastic Surgery News* 1987a). The joint statement recognized each other's right to practice within the boundaries of their specialty and their inevitable overlap in some areas of practice. It affirmed that "Both societies do not accept, condone, or encourage statements improperly demeaning or disparaging other physicians or groups of physicians" and that "Both societies deplore . . . self-appointed champions of a specialty . . . making fraudulent or deceptive statements." Plastic surgeons inserted the statement that, until common parameters defining the length and scope of fellowship training are adopted, no fellowship can substitute for training in an approved residency program. Testimony at the congressional hearings provided ample evidence that the joint statement on intraprofessional relations did not end the turf battle. The hearings, nevertheless, highlighted the need to tone down the conflict. It was bad publicity for all involved.

The ASPRS requested a meeting with the American Academy of Dermatology in 1990 to discuss advertising (*Plastic Surgery News,* 1990b). The ASPRS leaders argued that when dermatologists advertise cosmetic surgery and mention they are board certified without naming their board, prospective patients assume they are board-certified plastic surgeons. Although the two groups reached no resolution on that issue, they agreed to work together to stop unqualified practitioners from doing chemical peels and to work to require accreditation of office facilities. Over the next three years the ASPRS participated in an AMA-sponsored ad hoc committee on advertising guidelines with the American Academy of Dermatology, the American Academy of Facial Plastic and Reconstructive Surgery, and the American Academy of Otolaryngology (*Plastic Surgery News* 1994a). The FTC required the committee to "fence in" language about the criteria for authoritative board certification in its proposed guidelines. As a result, neither the ASPRS nor the American Board of Medical Specialties supported the final section of the guidelines on listing board certification.

Like the AMA, the American Board of Medical Specialties also pressured plastic surgeons to end their turf battles with other specialties. In the late 1980s it asked the American Board of Plastic Surgery and the American Board of Otolaryngology to explore a "horizontal pathway" to joint certification of a subspecialty in head and neck plastic and reconstructive surgery (*Plastic Surgery News* 1997c). The two specialties came to the brink of an agreement in 1995. They sponsored a joint symposium that year to develop a consensus statement about what is the state of the art in head and neck plastic surgery *Plastic Surgery News* 1995b). The negotiations broke down when plastic surgeons removed all references in the negotiated agreement to "jointly" conferring and awarding certification in plastic surgery within the head and neck region (Neale 1996). Otolaryngologists then balked, claiming that the plastic surgeons had reneged once again.

Repeatedly faced with stalled negotiations, the American Board of Otolaryngology applied several times to the American Board of Medical Specialties for a certificate of added qualifications in facial plastic and reconstructive surgery. This certificate could be granted unilaterally by the otolaryngologists' own board after an applicant completed requirements. Such a certificate ignores the authority of the American Board of Plastic Surgery in this area of medicine. As a result, it would likely accelerate the new trend for states to declare certification by boards not recognized by the American Board of Medical Specialties, such as the American Board of Facial Plastic and Reconstructive Surgery, as substantially equivalent to the umbrella organization's own boards. This trend undermines the legitimacy of the American Board of Medical Specialties.

Once again the American Board of Medical Specialties pleaded with its two boards in 1997 to resume discussions on a horizontal pathway to certification of plastic surgery within the head and neck region, certification that would preserve the authority of both existing boards. The two specialties' associations sponsored a second joint symposium that year on aesthetic and reconstructive rhinoplasty (*Plastic Surgery News* 1997e). The success of that symposium held promise for a future accord. In early 1998 the two boards signed a resolution adopted by the American Board of Medical Specialties. The resolution declared that they would develop a joint subcertification in plastic surgery within the head and neck region. The American Academy of Facial Plastic and Reconstructive Surgery and its self-designated certification board opposed the resolution. They objected because they had already developed a fellowship training program and a structure for independent board certification for otolaryngologists (Adamson 1998). The president of the facial board questioned why otolaryngologists would want to work with the American Board of Plastic Surgery. He claimed the latter had stated it would use the program to control the numbers of otolaryngologists in cosmetic surgery. Despite the facial board's concerns, negotiations between the American Board of Otolaryngology and the American Board of Plastic Surgery are ongoing at this time (American Board of Otolaryngology, 1999, personal communication; American Board of Plastic Surgery, 1999, personal communication). There may be a treaty in the future.

Board-certified plastic surgeons have so far failed to stop other physicians from encroaching on their cosmetic turf. As a result, they have resorted to more aggressive marketing, the subject of the next two chapters. Whether they realize it or not, plastic surgeons have followed the advice of their old nemesis, Jack Anderson. In 1987 he published an editorial about the plastic surgery controversy that asked, "Why the Fuss?" Based on readers' responses to a *Psychology Today* survey, he estimated that it would take six thousand practitioners twenty years to fix all the noses that Americans did not like. That would still leave them 60 million complexions, 30 million chins, 6 million eyes, etc. This is not the place to point out the problems with his methodology. Despite the errors of his estimates, his main point holds: "There are more than enough cosmetic facial surgery patients for everyone." He urged all practitioners interested in cosmetic surgery to work together. He suggested that "funds could be pooled to educate the public regarding the virtues of cosmetic surgery, thereby stimulating demand. . . . An impossible dream? Not for men of good will who see the big picture" (Anderson 1987, 709). Detente was not necessary for most practitioners of cosmetic surgery to see the big picture of commercialism, as the next chapter reveals.

Turf Battles, Fragmentation, and the Threat to Professional Authority

Cosmetic surgery is not the only contested area of medical practice. General practitioners were driven out of childbirth by obstetricians. Orthopedists and neurosurgeons dispute each other's claim to the spinal column. Radiologists must defend their new technologies against seizure by other specialists. Twenty-three medical societies recently protested the mandatory use of hospitalists by some managed care programs (Foubister 1999). There is even a turf battle brewing between the AMA and the American Board of Medical Specialties over who has the authority and responsibility to provide the continuing assessment of physician competence now demanded by hospitals, managed care plans, insurance companies, and the public (Prager 1999).

Turf battles have a long history in medicine. Their widespread prevalence and high visibility in the nineteenth century were major obstacles to public acceptance of medical authority. The AMA achieved power in part by gathering into one occupation the middle- and upper-class male practitioners who embraced germ theory and eschewed commercialism. Presenting a unified front was an important strategy for achieving public recognition of their authority in health care. It also lent legitimacy to their campaign to exclude, limit, and subordinate their competitors. To maintain this cohesion, regular physicians had to refrain from publicly criticizing each other. This code of silence became so ingrained that physicians have since been chastised for not adequately policing their colleagues. Silence about disagreements also kept most turf battles civil and hidden from public view. But, there have always been concerns about competition within the profession.

Much of the concern about competition has centered on medicine's transformation over the last fifty years from a profession dominated by general practitioners to one of specialists and subspecialists. Some charge that specialization, formalized by board certification, is nothing more than an economic weapon to limit competition in a clinical area (Walt 1986). Specialization is also criticized for splintering medical school curriculums, undermining the quality of general training, and de-skilling medical practitioners. Scientific studies that demonstrate better outcomes by board-certified specialists compared to generalists are rarely undertaken. Board certification, nevertheless, has much face value. It appeals to modern society's respect for rigorous training, reductionism, and the concept of expertise. Despite the AMA's policy to the contrary, board certification is treated as a de facto specialty license by hospitals, managed care programs, and insurance companies. The increasingly common requirement for board certification makes it difficult for others to enter an area of noncommercial practice claimed by a specialty. The requirement also allows relatively inexperienced, but board-certified, practitioners to displace more experienced practitioners without similar certification. Just as board-certified specialists can use their claims of expertise to displace generalists, subspecialists can use their reputed additional expertise to displace those who are merely specialists. When physicians in danger of being displaced defend their economic interests, territorial skirmishes result.

Many have commented that specialization intellectually and functionally pulls physicians apart. Differentiation of interests and work tasks creates a division of labor within the profession. It is a mistake, however, to think of this division of labor as immutable and a mistake to think of specialties as separate pieces of the larger professional pie. Neither illness nor medical innovation recognize or honor the boundaries of man-made specialties. New theories, technologies, and clinical approaches constantly emerge that cut across the boundaries of the twenty-four specialty boards and the seventy-five subspecialties now recognized by the American Board of Medical Specialties. Moreover, changes in social, economic, and political institutions lead to changes in the organization and tasks of practitioners. On a macro level, for example, the commercialization of medical products and services and corporatization of service delivery have enlarged the roles of physician researchers and physician administrators and truncated the roles of many rank-and-file practitioners. On a micro level, these changes have made elective procedures that are paid for out of pocket, such as cosmetic surgery, an attractive area of practice to all types of specialists facing intense competition in their narrow specialty. The limited demand for some specialties, therefore, not only pulls physicians apart, it sometimes pushes segments back together.

Rosemary Stevens (1999) suggests that an "expansionary network model" may be more appropriate than a pie model to describe the evolving structure of the medical profession. It recognizes the proliferation of links and overlaps between subspecialties and the existence of hybrid specialities created by double-boarding. It also could recognize the links between rank-and-file practitioners and physicians in academic, administrative, and organizational leadership roles, links that Eliot Freidson argues are significant and usually overlooked (1989). A network model assumes that the connections are recognized by members of the profession as valuable because they bind the diverse segments of the medical profession into a more powerful social entity. Alternatively, if the connections are regarded as competitive encroachment, they will create contested jurisdictions.

Andrew Abbott (1988) reveals that contested jurisdictions typify the interdependent system (e.g., network) of professions that controls expert knowledge, whether it be medical, legal, accounting, or another field. He documents that professions sometimes flourish, sometimes fuse, sometimes fragment, and sometimes fail. Faced with external and internal changes, they are never static. His competition model applies as much to intraprofessional relations, such as between medical specialties, as to interprofessional relations. The history of the learned professions offers a caution for medical specialties and subspecialties engaged in turf battles. If a truce cannot be reached, balkanization may result. The more public and more acrimonious the conflicts are, the more potential they have to destroy the cohesion that transformed the medical profession into arguably the most powerful occupation in America by the middle of the twentieth century. Physician authority is at risk of collateral damage when turf wars rage.

6 | Caveat Emptor
Selling Surgery

Commercialism has become synonymous with American life. The nineteenth-century industrial transformation not only increased labor productivity and available goods, it also put more disposable income in the hands of the general public. Everyone from merchants to ministers sought a share of the new disposable income. Medical practitioners were no different. They multiplied in the unregulated market, hawking everything from herbal and magnetic cures to hydropathy and spinal adjustments. In the absence of much scientific research on treatment outcomes, practitioners were free to make grandiose claims about the efficacy of their treatments. Many aggressively solicited patients. Most relied on advertisements, speaking engagements, books, testimonials, and media publicity in their local area to generate business. Like the early twentieth-century beauty doctors discussed in chapter 3, some attracted publicity with theatrical performances of surgical, electrical, or other treatments. Others took their show on the road and used circus, vaudeville, and theater performers to attract an audience, as well as shills, alcohol, and addictive substances to stimulate sales of their patent medicines (McNamara 1995). The motto painted on the porch of the original Palmer School of chiropractic medicine in Iowa summed up the view of many practitioners in this competitive, commercial market: "Early to bed, early to rise, work like hell, and advertise." As chiropractor

B. J. Palmer added in his 1926 book, *Selling Yourself,* "Only the mints can make money without advertising."

This chapter reviews the changing policies for marketing medical care. A discussion of the content of several hundred cosmetic surgery advertisements published in Yellow Pages, metropolitan newspapers, and state and local magazines from around the country follows. Although not a scientifically representative sample of all printed advertisements published in the early and late 1990s, the range of content and styles of presentation are illustrated. The roles of the American Society of Plastic and Reconstructive Surgeons (ASPRS), marketing firms, and finance companies are examined. The chapter concludes with a discussion of the spread of commercialization in cosmetic surgery.

Marketing Policies

Central to the American Medical Association's struggle for organization, cultural legitimacy, professional authority, and autonomy in the decades surrounding the turn of the twentieth century was the campaign to drive the quacks out of medicine. This was more than just a desire by allopathic physicians to reduce competition for patients by irregulars with different disease theories and treatments. The American Medical Association (AMA) eventually absorbed many eclectics and homeopaths willing to embrace germ theory and a scientific foundation for medicine. At the same time, it excluded others—including some who adhered to the allopathic philosophy of medicine. It also was more than an attempt to restrict medical practice to those with adequate training. At the time, few practicing physicians, including AMA members, had graduated from one of the only three medical schools judged to be adequate by Abraham Flexner in his 1910 report to the Carnegie Foundation. Nor could it be explained by outcomes because bad outcomes were endemic in the days before blood transfusions, antibiotics, and chemotherapies. As discussed in chapter 3, the distinction between regular and irregular practitioners using plastic techniques in surgery rested in large part on the extent to which their medical practice was commercial. Those who advertised or sought personal publicity in other ways to solicit patients were most likely to be targeted as quacks. Turn-of-the-century AMA leaders believed that blatantly commercial medicine would undermine their campaign for professional privileges and status.

The AMA formally banned advertising and other forms of solicitation in its first code of ethics in 1847: "It is derogatory to the dignity of the profession, to resort to public advertisements or private cards or handbills, inviting the attention in individuals affected with particular diseases . . . to boast of cures and remedies,—to adduce certificates of skill and success, or to perform any other similar acts" (qtd. in Olson 1990, 353). The American College of Surgeons, established in 1913, required members additionally to pledge to "shun unwarranted publicity, dishonest moneyseeking and commercialism as disgraceful to our profession" (Hugo 1997). State medical societies adopted similar bans. The 1920 Massachusetts Medical Society Code of Ethics elaborated: "A spirit of competition considered honorable in purely business transactions cannot exist among physicians without diminishing their usefulness and lowering the dignity and standing of the profession" (Massachusetts Medical Society 1961).

Commercialism threatened the AMA's efforts to convince the public that medicine was not a commodity or a trade. Instead, the AMA argued that the institution of medicine was a special service with a fiduciary interest in the well-being of patients. Patients could not be consumers because the new, evolving, medical science that promised better outcomes was too complex for lay persons to understand. They had to depend on the knowledge, skills, and compassion of their physicians when they were sick, and trust the AMA to ensure that their physicians were trained in the latest scientific knowledge.

Establishing this service ethic was crucial to organized medicine's bid for recognition as a profession. A profession is an occupation granted special privileges because of its special responsibilities. The special privileges that these physicians wanted included restrictive licensure to guarantee a monopoly over their work and the autonomy to define the boundaries, qualifications, and standards of their work, free from outside regulation. In return the AMA pledged to protect the public's interest and ensure physician competency through peer oversight.

The exact wording of the AMA ban on advertising changed several times after the turn of the century. More specific prohibitions regarding solicitation were added until it was streamlined in 1957. From then until 1976 it read simply, "He [the physician] should not solicit patients." The AMA's Judicial Council made it clear what this statement meant. "The practice of medicine should not be commercialized or treated as a commodity in trade. Respecting the dignity of their calling, physicians should resort only to the most limited use of advertising and then only to the extent necessary to serve the common good and improve the health of mankind" (American Medical Association 1971, 27). The council defined solicitation as attempts to obtain patients by "persuasion or influence," including implied or overt self-laudatory claims of superior medical skills and inflated expectations of medical outcomes, testimonials, and advertising. Only discreet announcements of name, type of practice, location, and office hours were allowed. Physicians who violated the rules were subjected to strong sanctions. They would be expelled from local medical associations, ending referrals from other members. They would be denied hospital privileges. They also could be assessed financial penalties and could have their licenses to practice medicine suspended

Sociologists and economists argue that professional gatekeeping such as accreditation of training programs, licensure, specialty certification, and advertising bans protect the interests of the professionals more than the interests of the public. At least in theory, they should reduce potentially divisive conflict among colleagues within the profession (Freidson 1989) and the potential for turf wars between professions (Abbot 1988). They also should hinder the development of alternative therapies (Cox and Foster 1990). In reality, they inflate medical care costs because they reduce competition and restrict consumer knowledge (Gross 1984). Moreover, they fail to ensure professional competence because physicians have proven to be reluctant to judge the practice of colleagues (Freidson 1980).

Advertising bans by an organized profession such as medicine also violate the 1890 Sherman Act that declared any restraint of trade or commerce by a "combination" is illegal. The Supreme Court, however, originally interpreted the law to apply only to private entities. The Court continues to recognize states' rights to enact laws, such as restrictive licensure for the public good, even when these laws restrain trade or commerce. The same holds true for activities of the federal government. Bans against advertising (and other anticompetitive practices, such as adoption of a minimum fee schedule) by private professional organizations would not be protected by the states' rights doctrine. Nevertheless, these private restraints of trade by high-status professions, such as law and medicine, went unchallenged until the 1970s. Justice Story set the precedent in 1834 when he explicitly excluded those "in the learned professions" in his definition of trade (cited in Freidson 1986, 116). His qualification was reaffirmed in a 1932 Supreme Court case that declared other services, such as cleaners, subject to the antitrust law, and again in a 1949 ruling on real-estate services. In contrast, the Court upheld a ban on advertising by Oregon dentists in 1935 because dentistry was "a profession treating bodily ills and demanding different standards of conduct from those which are traditional in the competition of the market place"(116).

The cultural climate and the Supreme Court's perspective changed by 1975. That year the Court struck down the Virginia State Bar's minimum fee schedule for the routine services of lawyers. The Court did not intend its ruling to end the special treatment of the learned professions. The ruling contained the caveat that "it would be unrealistic to view the practice of professions as interchangeable with other business activities and automatically to apply to the professions antitrust concepts which originated in other areas" (qtd. in Freidson 1986, 117). Nevertheless, the next year the Court struck down bans on advertising prices by the Virginia Pharmacy Board and subsequently the State Bar of Arizona on First Amendment grounds of free commercial speech. In the first case the Court explicitly noted that the state had the right to license pharmacists and eliminate competition from others who did not meet the state's licensure criteria to protect the public interest, but it could not deny information about price differences among licensed pharmacists to the public. The ruling again suggested that the Court might have a different opinion if other professions were involved, and the chief justice asserted that services offered by lawyers and doctors may not be as routinized as the prepackaged drugs involved in this case. The second case was decided by a five-to-four vote. Dissenting justices argued that legal services were rarely, if ever, so routine that they could be equated with prepackaged drugs and opposed lifting bans on advertising prices of any legal work. The majority ruling reiterated the caveat made in the pharmacy case and affirmed that some kinds of advertising may warrant restrictions, but not the price of the "routine" legal services involved in this case.

Although the Court appeared to be open to maintaining a distinction between the learned professions and other service providers under antitrust law, the camel's nose was under the tent. The public was growing less enamored with lawyers and doctors, who seemed to be proliferating and prospering in the severe recession of the 1970s. The legal profession became the politically correct target of jokes about greed and ethics. Medical malpractice suits were rising rapidly, reflecting an erosion of trust in the doctor-patient relationship. Some consumer groups publicly challenged the altruistic claims and authority of physicians. Health care costs were at the forefront of an inflationary spiral that was undermining both private and public spending power. The federal government wanted to rein in health care spending.

Recognizing the direction of change, the Federal Trade Commission (FTC) issued an antitrust complaint in 1975 against the AMA and two professional medical organizations in Connecticut for their bans against "soliciting business, by advertising or otherwise" (Federal Trade Commission 1975, 2). The FTC challenged not only the AMA's restrictions on dissemination of price information, but also its ban on solicitation of patients. The commission concluded in 1978 that the AMA's suppression of truthful advertising by physicians was a violation of the Sherman Act (Federal Trade Commission 1997, 3, 14). A split Supreme Court in 1982 left intact a 1980 federal appeals court ruling in favor of the FTC.

Following the Court's ruling, the AMA led a campaign for federal legislation to exempt state-regulated professions such as medicine from the jurisdiction of the FTC. It won a moratorium on FTC enforcement when a majority of representatives in the House agreed to cosponsor the bill. The reprieve proved temporary. Media investigations of campaign contributions by the health industry's political action committees raised public concern about whose interests the AMA wanted to protect—the profession's or the public's (Feldstein 1996, 150). The Reagan administration, many business leaders, and other health and consumer organizations opposed the bill. Feeling the pressure, the Senate defeated the bill.

Under the broad order issued by the FTC, the AMA now can prohibit only false and deceptive advertisements. The American Dental Association was forced to sign a consent order that same year, saying it would not restrict its members from truthfully advertising or soliciting business. Similar consents were signed by associations of other kinds of health workers, including the American Psychological Association and the National Association of Social Workers. Attempts by these two organizations to prohibit members from participating in patient-referral services and using patient testimonials also were stopped, although the FTC allows them to restrict testimonials from patients vulnerable to influence and to ban testimonials from current psychotherapy patients.

A flurry of additional consent orders followed attempts by other state and national associations and state regulatory boards to restrict aspects of advertising by health care workers. Taken together, these consent orders prohibited associations and state boards from banning advertisements of training, experience, services, fees, financing terms, acceptance of Medicare and credit cards, and foreign language skills. Nor may they ban offers of free services, discounts, guarantees, claims of special expertise and superiority, and listings of products, such as contact lenses, for sale. The consent orders also prohibited associations and state boards from limiting the amount, duration, and size of advertising announcements and requiring advertisements to be in "good taste" or to be submitted for review before use. Attempts to regulate taste, such as the Michigan Optometric Association's prohibition against the use of large signs or lettering and representations of eyes, eyeglasses, or the human head, were deemed illegal along with the Massachusetts Board of Registration in Optometry's prohibition against "sensational advertisements." The AMA now expressly allows all forms of advertising that are not deceptive: "A physician may publicize himself as a physician through any commercial publicity or other form of public communication (including any newspaper, magazine, telephone directory, radio, television, direct mail or other advertising) provided that the communication shall not be misleading because of the omission of necessary material information, shall not contain any false or misleading statement, or shall not otherwise operate to deceive" (qtd. in Olson 1990, 354).

The Practice Builders

The FTC's actions paved the way for the reentry of overt commercialism in medicine. Prior to the new policy, existing marketing efforts were necessarily indirect and subtle. Physicians had to avoid appearing to solicit patients through self-aggrandizement. They could unobtrusively court referrals from primary practitioners and previous patients, seek positions on medical school faculties, publish books and articles, give lectures, and, if asked, respond to reporters' inquiries about treatments. Although time-consuming, all were effective ways to establish a reputation as an expert, if not the "best" or "greatest" in the field. Some found it more efficient and less chancy to hire public relations consultants to put their names in front of the public, although most physicians considered using them to be unethical. The FTC's new policy not only ended the secrecy about these relationships, it also legalized obvious solicitation. One New York City firm that only started representing physicians in 1992 signed up some eight hundred by 1998, billing them about six million dollars annually

(Glabman 1998). An author in the plastic surgeons' official journal complained, "Plastic surgery is entering the era of merchandising. One need only turn pages in national women's magazines or such regional periodicals as *New York* or *Far West* to see the handiwork of the PR men" (Rubin 1982, 117). While he correctly predicted that plastic surgeons would soon "give lectures to the laity in department stores," he did not anticipate that his own professional organization would cosponsor them six years later (*Plastic Surgery News* 1988b, 2).

The first paid advertisements for cosmetic surgery appeared in the late 1970s. Leaders of the ASPRS warned members against "hucksterism," "worshipping the golden calf," and succumbing to "the siren song of instant riches." Most board-certified plastic surgeons resisted advertising at first. A few California practitioners, however, began advertising on television and radio and in the print media. Among them were plastic surgeons. A 1977 editorial in *Plastic and Reconstructive Surgery* asked, "What can certification by ABPS [American Board of Plastic Surgery] . . . mean to the public if physicians (even a few) are willing to prostitute themselves and their profession by participating in such ethical cesspools" (Webster 1977, 100).

As the number who hired public relations firms and advertising agencies increased, the marketing of cosmetic surgery grew and the editorial rhetoric became more shrill. A 1980 editorial claimed that "unscrupulous borderline sociopaths are crawling out of the walls to get their share of the 'action'" and "some of our respected peers and elders have turned out to be closet hustlers" (Gorney 1980, 752). This ASPRS leader was incensed that some of his colleagues used their board certification in plastic surgery as a "commercial logo," a practice that has since become an ASPRS recommendation. Leaders of the ASPRS's sister organization, the American Society for Aesthetic Plastic Surgery, reacted similarly to the FTC's policy. The 1981 presidential address was a diatribe against advertising. Despite the FTC ruling, the president warned members that the organization's code of ethics did not permit advertising that encourages or solicits cosmetic treatments (Kaye 1981). The Supreme Court's decision a year later ended all hope the leaders of plastic surgery associations had of persuading members of their specialty to voluntarily adhere to traditional ethics when competitors from other specialties were free to advertise and call themselves cosmetic surgeons or facial plastic surgeons. By 1988 a survey indicated that 48 percent of board-certified plastic surgeons advertised in the Yellow Pages and some advertised in newspapers, magazines, direct mail, television, and radio, as did many of their competitors for cosmetic surgery (*Plastic Surgery News* 1989c). An ASPRS leader was moved to comment, "The field of elective aesthetic surgery now resembles the midway of a cheap carnival, complete with flashing colored lights, gaudy trappings, and loud barkers" (Gorney 1989a, 800).

His charge was an exaggeration, but advertising quickly became the norm, and a small segment of it was in dubious taste for professionals. Some print-media editors banned before-and-after ads because they found them offensive. The most infamous ad of the 1980s, however, was not a before-and-after. It was an arresting photograph of "a brunet bombshell in a white bathing suit and silver spike heels [who] stands, chest thrust forward, next to a bright red sports car" (Hughes 1988, 1). The copy above her read, "Automobile by Ferrari. Body by Forshan." The eighty thousand dollar ad in the *Los Angeles* magazine generated considerable controversy because Dr. Forshan had not operated on the model, raising questions about deception in addition to poor taste. The irony of the subsequent revelation that another cosmetic surgeon had operated on Forshan's model was not lost on the media. That same year another doctor issued a press release which included a picture of him standing next to Miss San Diego and the announcement that he was the "official facial plastic surgery consultant" for the Miss San Diego beauty contest. His patient, pageant officials, and most other physicians were perturbed by his public relations effort. Some other marketing attempts were equally disturbing. A video sent to prospective patients by a group of physicians featured comedian Phyllis Diller in a green wig advising, "Don't ever go to a doctor who operates in a Ford van." Perhaps the most ill-advised press kit of the decade included test tubes of greasy, yellow chicken fat that a public relations firm thought would generate favorable stories on liposuction featuring its two clients as experts (Garfield 1987, 40). The ASPRS campaign for legislated advertising restrictions, discussed in the previous chapter, fared no better at eliminating questionable marketing strategies than efforts to promote voluntary compliance with traditional ethics.

ASPRS National Advertising

Frustrated by their inability to prevent such advertising, ASPRS leaders reversed direction and tried to guide the content of members' advertising by offering a "Marketing Your Practice" workshop in 1985 (*Plastic Surgery News* 1985). Many members welcomed the two-day program, which became a regular event. Within a year the society established a separate marketing department charged with helping individual members compete in the new medical marketplace as well as strategically marketing the specialty of plastic surgery to the general public. As discussed in chapter 4, this department developed numerous services and products for members to use and worked aggressively to promote a favorable public image for the specialty.

In 1997 the ASPRS Marketing Department had a million dollar budget for the largest marketing campaign in the history of ASPRS (Stott 1997a). Some of the old-guard plastic surgeons who vehemently opposed the commercialization of cosmetic surgery in the 1970s and 1980s must have been outraged by the ads. In one an attractive woman wearing a cleavage-revealing swimsuit says, "I could have worn padded swimsuits. I could have learned to live with what I had. I had breast enlargement surgery instead." In another a man says, "I could have worn baggy T-shirts to the beach. I could have laughed at the 'love handle' jokes. I had liposuction instead." The ASPRS went from condemning commercial ads at the 1989 congressional hearings on cosmetic surgery to sponsoring them in less than a decade. Talking about the campaign, the 1997 president of the ASPRS acknowledged, "Ten years ago, it would have been grounds for impeachment" (*Plastic Surgery News* 1997a, 1).

The campaign had similar full-page ads for eyelid surgery and facelifts, ads that also used real patients between thirty and fifty. The ads appeared in five women's magazines and two men's magazines, in an ASPRS-sponsored educational insert in *USA Today* at the time of the national meeting, and on television during *Lifetime* and CNN segments. All contained statements like the one for breast enlargement. "If you're considering breast enlargement surgery the American Society of Plastic and Reconstructive Surgeons wants to help you make the right decision. One that can raise your confidence. One that can improve the way you feel about yourself. Call . . . for a list of our surgeons in your area." The society's logo and website address also appear. A sidebar warns readers and viewers to use a well-trained, qualified, experienced surgeon and informs them that ASPRS members are trained to perform both cosmetic and reconstructive plastic surgery. It concludes, "In other words, the same plastic surgeon who does a child's cleft palate or rebuilds a woman's breast lost to mastectomy is also trained in cosmetic procedures—such as liposuction, breast enlargement, eyelid surgery and facelifts."

The ASPRS made the ads available to regional societies for use in local publications and electronic media and offered in-office displays to members. *Plastic Surgery News* advised members to integrate their local marketing with the society's national campaign (*Plastic Surgery News* 1997d). It suggested members employ a public relations firm to work with the local press, arrange seminars, speak to professional or community groups, and write opinion columns for local papers on where cosmetic surgery and reconstructive surgery fit into health care. The article also reassured members that the country's demographics are ideal for cosmetic surgery. An estimated five to six million are in the target market of individuals thirty-five to fifty-four years of age who are favorably disposed to have cosmetic surgery.

Targeting the market for cosmetic surgery is one of the reasons given for the national marketing campaign in a related article in the same issue (Stott 1997b). The other is the need to control the public message about the society and its members. Using the language of commercial marketing, the author says the principles of selling surgery are the same as those for selling paper towels, although the consumer decision is a long-term process, like buying an expensive automobile, which necessitates continuous marketing. For these reasons the ASPRS decided to extend the campaign. Its ads for 2000 were posted on its Internet site.

Marketing Firms

About the same time the ASPRS established its Marketing Department, ads for private marketing companies appeared in *Plastic Surgery News*. Most of these companies specialize in the niche market of "discretionary-oriented health care services," another way of saying commercial medical services. These same companies advertise in publications of otolaryngologists and other competitors in the cosmetic surgery market. Some conduct symposia around the country on how to build a "two-million dollar cosmetic surgery practice" by "implementing proven promotional systems and techniques" which include marketing auxiliary services such as spas and laser hair removal and skin care. Attendance at a one- or two-day symposium in 2000 cost a physician around one thousand dollars, and more if an office manager also attends, but this is only the initial outlay. Custom consultation and advertising are expensive.

Full-service marketing companies offer both public relations and advertising services. According to their ads, they can assess a current practice, train staff to sell services, develop a marketing plan, provide support services for that plan, coach the physician for media appearances, make contacts with local media, track results, and conduct patient-satisfaction surveys, all for separate fees or as part of a package of services. There are additional fees to use the support services, which consist of designing and placing ads in Yellow Pages and in print and electronic media; developing other promotional strategies, such as conducting local seminars or writing an advice column for a local paper; and materials such as brochures, patient newsletters, and videotapes. The website of one of these companies in the summer of 1999 contained a copy of an article by the CEO in which he tells prospective physician clients that they should be prepared to spend $150,000 or more to build and maintain a $1.5 million cosmetic surgery practice, excluding the income they can derive from using an in-office surgical facility. He also suggests using referral companies that advertise cosmetic surgery and funnel prospective patients to physicians for a fee. Some marketing companies offer packaged marketing plans that reduce the costs by using the same or similar ads and materials for physicians in different states. Freelancers usually charge less than agencies. Physicians also can develop their own marketing plans and materials, but they cannot escape some significant costs if they want to advertise.

Yellow Pages

Cosmetic surgery is advertised in most, if not all, metropolitan areas as well as many smaller cities. Yellow Pages in Sunbelt metropolitan areas usually contain many pages of display ads in addition to the free two- or three-line listings and the less expensive, expanded in-column ads. The 1998–1999 Phoenix area book, for example, contained three and one-half pages of display ads at the beginning of the "Physicians and Surgeons—Medical and Osteopathic" general listing, more than twelve pages under the self-designated specialty listing for "Surgery, Plastic and Reconstructive," and five pages under "Dermatology." In contrast, the Boston Yellow Pages contained only about six pages of cosmetic surgery ads and physician listings.

Where telephone listings for cosmetic surgery are numerous, they must compete for the reader's attention. In these markets, many physicians buy ads and place them in multiple directories or in more than one place in the same directory. Some pay extra for color or other special features. Artistic graphics, illustrations, borders, font size and type, and boldface print are used liberally to make an ad stand out. Pictures of the physician, usually male, are common, along with an occasional picture of an "actual patient," usually female. The cost can be substantial. A full-page, full-color ad in the 1999 Phoenix or Los Angeles Yellow Pages cost more than six thousand dollars per month over the twelve month duration of the ad. Without color or other special features, a full-page ad still cost more than four thousand dollars per month in these markets. Smaller ads cost proportionately less.

The display ads vary widely in style in the Yellow Pages examined in eight cities. A few are discreet announcements of a physician or hospital name, specialty, and location—not much different than what would have been permitted under the AMA's old code of ethics. A few have pictures of patients that look like they belong in a "girlie" magazine and self-aggrandizing claims such as "Rated one of the 'Top Docs' 1996 & 1997 in . . . Magazine Survey," "Listed in 'The Best Doctors in . . . ,'" "As Seen on TV," or "Simply the Finest Cosmetic Surgery Money Can Buy." Most are in between these extremes.

Yellow Pages ads typically include a list of cosmetic procedures, statements about board certification, and membership in professional associations along with their trademarks. More often than not the certifying board is mentioned, whether or not it is recognized by the American Board of Medical Specialties. Although not as common, many of the ads include years of surgical experience, offers of free consultation and brochures, use of video-imaging, financing, private surgical facilities, personal Internet addresses, and the ASPRS Internet address. More rarely, hospital or medical school affiliation is noted. A few contain warnings that not all cosmetic surgeons are the same. For example, one ad mentions that training can range from a weekend to years of intensive study and experience. Another provides the telephone number of the American Board of Plastic Surgery and advises calling to see whether a physician is certified by that board or checking the local library's *Directory of Medical Specialists* under "Plastic Surgery." A few also stress that cosmetic surgery is "safer" and "more affordable than ever!" None of the ads in the directories examined contain information about the cost or the risk of complications.

Print-Media Ads

Some physicians use their Yellow Pages ads in local newspapers, tabloids, and magazines. Like Yellow Pages ads, print-media ads typically contain a list of cosmetic procedures, credentials, experience, professional associations, telephone numbers, and location, which can include more than one office. Offers of free consultations, brochures, videotapes, and use of video-imaging are common, as are association logos, financing, and Internet addresses in recent years. A few now mention that their surgical facilities are accredited. Besides new procedures, a rare mention of fees, and more ads for investor-owned facilities and referral services, there are no other differences in the cosmetic surgery ads that appeared in the beginning of the 1990s and those at the end of the decade.

There are some general differences between Yellow Pages ads and print-media ads. There is more artwork and more copy in the latter. Print-media ads are more likely to feature one procedure, although others may be listed. Some procedures, such as ear pinning, male breast reduction, abdominoplasty, and buttocks lifts, are rarely featured. There often is a caption to attract attention. Some stress ease or innovations (e.g., "LIPOSUCTION: A NEW BODY OVERNITE" and "UltraSonic Body Contouring: A Breakthrough in Fat Removal"). Others appeal to dominant cultural values such as control and youth (e.g., "ALL LIMITATIONS ARE SELF-IMPOSED," "Never Underestimate Your Power as a Woman," and "You *Can* Look Younger!"). Although not typical of print-media ads, there are more self-aggrandizing claims, such as "recently featured performing liposuction on Channel . . . News" or "a master of surgical artistry, renowned for great results." The latter was placed by a physician who had previously been suspended by his state medical board for poor patient care.

Pictures of physicians are much less common in print-media ads than in Yellow Pages ads. In contrast, pictures of patients, or models posing as patients, are much more common. The "patients" pictured or illustrated are, with rare exceptions, Anglo females, except in ads for hair-loss treatments. Only one of the several hundred ads examined had a picture of an African American woman. It appeared in a sixteen-page special advertising supplement to *the Washington Post Magazine* in 1996. Another ad mentions that a large proportion of patients are members of minority groups.

There appear to be large differences in the volume and content of print-media ads by area, although it has not been systematically studied. Boston has few ads, despite a high concentration of physicians. Smaller Midwestern cities such as Omaha and Milwaukee also appear to have relatively few. There are far more in Chicago and New York and still more in San Diego, Los Angeles, Phoenix, Denver, Dallas,

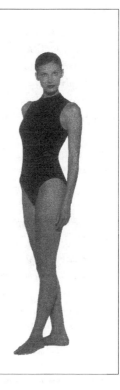

Beauty is a choice

and the choice is yours.

Are you ready to enhance your image,
raise your confidence,
enrich your life?

Then call for a private consultation with the
Cosmetic Surgery Specialist,

Dr. John Doe
Board Certified
(999) 999-9999

Financing Available

Figure 6.1. Composite ad

Washington, D.C., Palm Beach, and Miami. Ads in Sunbelt cities are more likely to be garish compared to ads in northern cities, although garish ads are in the small minority everywhere.

Most print-media ads are designed to fit the context in which they appear and the audience they target. Those in entertainment-oriented newspapers sometimes look like ads for topless bars with pictures of naked or nearly naked young women with big breasts and big hair, sometimes posed erotically. An ad in a gay publication offered discounts for patients associated with a service organization for people with AIDS. In contrast, those that appear in symphony programs and metro or state magazines that target an affluent segment of the population are generally more subdued and sometimes artistic. Botticelli's *Venus* and Da Vinci's *Vitruvian Man* appear in some ads. Renoir's *Dance at Bougival* is used in a Washington-area ad with the caption, "We've

Mastered The Fine Art Of Cosmetic Surgery." The fine art is marked with lines linking body parts to the names of cosmetic procedures surrounding the picture. Other ads feature original artwork. For example, three-quarters of a full-page ad in a 1997 *Texas Monthly* consists of a black-and-white, close-up picture of an elegant young woman in a formal dress with her hair pulled into a chignon, leaning back from her bent arm, which rests on a mirror that reflects her beautiful face. "INVITE COMPARISON" is the caption. Underneath the picture is the plastic surgeon's name in large print and seven short lines of small print that list his personal information. At the bottom of the page in very small print is a short list of procedures and a telephone number to request a brochure or private consultation. A facial plastic surgeon has a similarly artistic full-page ad in the same issue. A cropped black-and-white front view of a young woman's head and neck spans the page. Her hair also is pulled back. Only the lower half of her lovely face is lit. The small print copy, which reads like a *Vogue* cosmetic ad, frames the upper left quarter of her head and the lower right half of her face and neck. Among other things, the copy says that "a striking face can bedazzle, mesmerize . . . and launch a thousand ships" and claims that a gorgeous face can be made more beautiful through cosmetic surgery of the cheekbones, lips, and jawline. It suggests an improved self-image will come from the "amazing changes."

A small portion of ads take a humorous approach. A 1991 liposuction ad in the *Salt Lake City* magazine asks in big bold print, "A Little Too Hip?" A 1997 *New York* magazine ad shows a mermaid with her arms across her chest and copy that asks, "Are You Unhappy with What Mother Nature Gave You?" Another version of this ad in *Newsday* asks, "Wouldn't Beautiful Breasts Make Your Image Complete?" A 1996 eye surgery ad in the *Washington Post Magazine* suggests, "Take the trip of a lifetime . . . And leave your bags with us." A 1997 *Texas Monthly* ad for "male enhancement surgery" features Michelangelo's *David* with a leaf extending from his genital area to below his knees.

Although some editors ban them, before-and-after pictures are common. They can be disturbing, as demonstrated by a 1997 *Village Voice* liposuction ad that displays an overweight woman in a tiny bikini bottom holding her large breasts over her midriff folds and bulging abdomen. Or, they can be reasonably tasteful. A full-page layout of six procedures—four facial, one covered torso, and one covered buttocks—

in color on a black background fits the latter category. This ad has little copy beyond the standard personal information about the physician and the statement "Limousine Service" in smaller print. The same pictures appear enlarged in ads in other issues of the *San Diego Magazine* in 1991, ads that focus on only one procedure, but have more copy. The facelift ad has "After 48 Years" above the "before" picture, "After 3 Hours, 25 Minutes" above the "after" picture, and below the pictures, "It doesn't hurt to look good again. It doesn't cost much. And it sure doesn't take long."

Ads for new procedures, such as endoscopic breast implants and facial surgery or tumescent and ultrasonic liposuction, usually give a brief description of the procedure, emphasizing its advantages over previous procedures. Prospective patients who want more information are invited to call for brochures, videotapes, and appointments with consultants on the physician's staff or with the physician. Some ads are designed in a question-and-answer format to look like interviews with a physician. These typically have more information. Other ads announce community seminars on the new procedure or the more generic "latest advancements in cosmetic surgery." These seminars are sponsored by individual physicians, referral services, and hospitals. Hospitals find that ambulatory surgery on healthy individuals is a profitable use of their facilities.

Ads with more than the standard personal information about physicians, a reference to procedures, and offers of brochures or videotapes often make brief claims about cosmetic surgery's simplicity, safety, psychological benefits, or inexpensiveness, like the before-and-after ad already described. A few lack credibility with claims like "guaranteed painless procedures." Others contain warnings to check a physician's credentials and experience, similar to a few of the Yellow Pages ads, discussed previously.

Some ads for an institute, center, or clinic do not name a physician. In some cases these ads are for referral services. Occasionally this is suggested by a caption such as "All those plastic surgery ads . . . How do you separate fact from fiction?" In other cases the ads are for facilities owned by nonphysician investors who pay freelancing physicians by the procedure. Ads for these businesses have increased over the last decade despite many physicians' objections both to the idea of a secondary party profiting from their labor and to their emphasis on low prices.

Price information is rare, but it appears more frequently at the end of the 1990s than at the beginning. Using standard marketing strategies, a few ads announce vague discounts, such as "Sizzling Summer Specials." Others make the discount clear, a 10 percent reduction for Mother's Day or some other holiday, but say nothing about the base price. Very few mention specific costs. Among the exceptions is a 1997 *New York* magazine ad that announces in large print, "Look Like a Million For a Couple Of Thousand." Whether all or only some of the many procedures listed in this ad could be had for $2,000 and whether the cost of the surgical facility and anesthesia is included is unclear. Nevertheless, the ad conveys the idea that the cost of cosmetic surgery is within reach of middle-class individuals, who have proven that they are willing to spend that amount of money for discretionary items like a computer. A few of the cosmetic surgery ads by different doctors in a Phoenix-area entertainment-oriented newspaper in 1999 offer precise information for a list of procedures offered. The prices in one ad range from $1,495 for eyelid surgery to $4,795 for a facelift. One also offers a "Cash Discount Schedule" and financing.

Specific risks are not mentioned in ads, except indirectly and then only rarely. For example, a full-page ultrasonic liposuction ad in *Today's Arizona Woman* says that the doctor "feels his patients will have less bruising, swelling and discomfort" with the new procedure. Unspecified risks also are implied in warnings about choosing the "right" doctor. These warnings can read like "edvertising," a soft-sell approach that enhances the image of the doctor as an authority and educator performing a public service. In reality these ads are just another battlefield for the intraprofessional fight, covered in chapter 5. Most say that board certification in plastic and reconstructive surgery is the critical criterion for selecting a physician. One of the most elaborate examples notes the role of the American Board of Medical Specialties and its relation to the American Board of Plastic Surgery and compares a relatively detailed listing of the requirements of the American Board of Plastic Surgery with the "six month or 1 year plastic surgery (cosmetic surgery) specialty fellowship" of unnamed other doctors. In the likely event that prospective patients are confused about who these unnamed other doctors are, the copy notes, "There is no *authorized* [sic] ABMS certifying board called 'Cosmetic Surgery' or 'Facial Plastic and Reconstructive Surgery.'" The ad advises readers to call the American Board of Plastic Surgery or two referral services exclusively for board-certified plastic surgeons or visit the ASPRS website to check on a physician's credentials.

Complimentary Copy

The distinction between advertising and editorial content in small local publications is often blurred. Local magazines frequently provide supporting copy for advertisers, including cosmetic surgery advertisers. This "editorial" material emphasizes the value of appearance and presents cosmetic procedures in a positive light. It can take the form of editors' columns, health-advice columns, or articles. Regular advertisers sometimes appear as authors of articles or "Ask the Doctor about Cosmetic Surgery" columns.

Special advertising sections in larger publications also blur the distinction between advertising and editorial copy, like infomercials that appear on television. Although they look like regular news articles, the primary function of articles in special advertising sections is to reinforce the content of the surrounding ads. Those on cosmetic surgery usually quote extensively from press releases issued by the ASPRS and other specialty associations and from manufacturers of related medical products such as lasers or implants. Typical of most journalism, they mix in expert opinion and testimonials from previous patients. In prestigious publications like the *Washington Post* the commercial advertising nature of the text is identified. The text and ads are set off in a separate space, the pages are labeled "An Advertising Supplement," and a footnote at the end of the article says it was written by a freelance writer, not staff from the News Department. Nevertheless, readers could easily think that the articles were objective news copy. The commercial nature of at least some articles in local publications like *Valley Living* or *Scottsdale Magazine* is much less clear. These magazines appear to be primarily merchandising catalogs for local goods and professional services.

Community Presentations

The commercial nature of community seminars also is not always clear to participants. These presentations are a form of advertising that enhances physicians' authority and reputations at the same time that it markets their services. Information requested to make a "required" reservation to attend one of these free events is used for follow-up marketing efforts with announcements of other lecturers, new developments, brochures, patient newsletters, and telephone calls. Sometimes these presentations are hosted or cohosted by local television or radio stations that promote them in advance as a "community service."

The presentations typically discuss who is a good candidate for a procedure, what a procedure can realistically accomplish for a patient physically and psychologically, what the surgical experience will be like, some of the risks, and sometimes costs. There are always before-and-after pictures, a packet of written material to take home, and time to answer questions from the audience. The discussion of cost is usually left to staff, who also make laudatory comments about the physicians to reinforce their expertise to the audience.

Those sponsored by hospitals tend to be serious, formal presentations by staff and one or more physicians, with professionally produced slides and videotapes to illustrate their talks. Those sponsored by referral companies or physicians are not as formal, although they also use well-designed audiovisual materials. Sometimes the presenters represent different specialties, e.g., dermatology, otolaryngology, and plastic surgery. Other times there is only one presenter, the doctor hosting the seminar. Seminars for procedures like laser skin resurfacing may demonstrate the procedure on a real patient, reminiscent of early twentieth-century beauty doctor Crum, discussed in chapter 3. Hospitals are not as likely as individual physicians and referral services to stage demonstrations and offer gifts like complimentary cosmetic makeovers to attract an audience. They typically hand out health education materials. Refreshments and hors d'oeuvres are usually served.

A seminar sponsored by the Mayo Clinic in 1995 included a presentation on facelifts by a plastic surgeon who subsequently served as president of the ASPRS. More than most other presenters observed at this and other seminars, he focused on socializing the audience to have realistic expectations of risks and results. He urged prospective patients to weigh benefits against risks and gave specific examples of risks. He also gave examples of benefits, but warned that they are temporary. For example, he said it takes three to six months to see the full results of a facelift and then "the skin heads for the ground" again. He reinforced his point by pointing to the large number of third facelifts he does on patients, sometimes after only five or six years, although eight to twelve years is average. He advised the audience to be wary of heavily promoted new techniques, because past experience indicates that some will later be found to cause problems. Although the cautionary tone of his presentation verged on de-advertising, it created an aura of honesty that was likely to gain the trust of wavering prospective patients put off by more aggressive sales pitches, observed at other seminars, that downplayed risks. Based on questions, however, the audience members seemed more concerned about whether they could afford to have cosmetic surgery at such a prestigious facility than risks. By the 1990s, financing was available for patients who did not have the money on hand.

Financing

When the competition for cosmetic surgery patients increased, because of the changes discussed in chapter 4, and attempts by the ASPRS to reduce competition failed, the pool of patients had to be enlarged. No longer could most practitioners cater only to the elite who could afford to pay thousands of dollars in advance or the self-disciplined who saved the necessary money over time. They had to target a wider clientele. The social, psychological, and economic benefits of an attractive appearance, discussed in chapter 2, ensured that some would regard cosmetic surgery as an investment that could pay off in upward social mobility. Advertising and publicity provided the tool for recruiting this group. The only remaining obstacle was finding a way for cash-poor patients to pay for it.

Despite the rapid expansion of credit in the United States in the 1970s and 1980s, most cosmetic practitioners at that time were reluctant to accept credit cards or to arrange installment payments. If a patient defaults, there is nothing to repossess. Pursuing legal action is expensive and provides no assurance of eventual payment. Physicians express additional qualms about patients going into debt to pay for elective surgery. They worry that the larger the percentage of future income a patient commits to cosmetic surgery, the higher that patient's expectations will be about results, whether realistic or not. They worry that some will over-extend themselves and the resulting financial stress will undermine their satisfaction with their results. Worries notwithstanding, credit came to cosmetic surgery in the 1990s.

The first financing program specifically for cosmetic surgery was launched by the ASPRS in 1989. It pays physicians in advance. It does not require a physician to discount fees, nor does it involve much office work, and it takes no recourse against the physician if a patient defaults (*Plastic Surgery News* 1997g). The only problem with this bank-administered program is that applicants are screened carefully for credit worthiness. Approximately three-quarters are refused (Selz 1997).

Other companies have stepped in to fill the financing gap. Some buy individual financing contracts offered to patients by doctors. They arrange the payment schedule and set the annual interest rate. In 1998 it ranged from 9 percent for a patient with an excellent credit rating to 20 percent for one considered risky. If financed over three years, $5,000 in cosmetic surgery would cost a patient who qualifies for the 9 percent loan approximately $159 per month and yield $724 in interest payments to the finance company, plus additional fees in some cases. A patient with a poor credit rating would pay $185 per month and a total of $1,189 in interest to the finance company willing to take the risk for a 20 percent return.

Other finance companies, like investor-owned facilities, have positioned themselves as middlemen between the pool of prospective patients and physicians. They assume the financial burden of advertising and aggressively use print media, radio, and television to recruit prospective patients. The finance companies refer those they choose to finance to physicians who are under contract to provide medical services at a discount in return for the additional business. The ads emphasize that cosmetic surgery is no longer only for the rich and famous; it is now available for no money down and low weekly or monthly payments.

Jayhawk Acceptance's entry into the cosmetic surgery referral business attracted front-page attention in the *Wall Street Journal* (Selz 1997). The used-car financing company, which built its business by targeting marginal borrowers, had emerged from bankruptcy and believed it had the right experience to "capitalize on America's vanity." The company's goal is to do for cosmetic surgery "what GMAC financing did for automobiles," which was to make them available to most Americans (Barry 1998). The company arranged ten thousand surgeries in its first two years. Jayhawk's president describes the typical credit patient as a woman approaching thirty who earns in the high $20,000s and sees cosmetic surgery as an "investment." Some have only a "C" credit rating. He estimates that the credit market for cosmetic surgery could be four or five times the size of the cash market. He may be right. The president of another financing company claims that his three-year-old referral service schedules an average of four hundred to five hundred cosmetic surgeries each month, and the majority of the patients were not actively shopping for cosmetic surgery when they saw the company's television commercial. Their commercial dangles the prospect that a viewer can be the person he or she always wanted to be for no money down and payments as low as $38 a week.

To provide some protection from the expected higher default rate with its marginal borrowers, Jayhawk charges physicians a one-time fee of $900 and routinely holds back 40 percent of their payment until the money is recovered from the borrower—a practice that physicians do not like. Many physicians object in principle to a financing company operating as a medical referral service. They believe that these companies will do to uninsured elective surgery what managed care has done to the rest of medicine by controlling access to patients and dictating cost-efficient treatments and wage concessions. In contrast, Jayhawk's president argues that physicians who object to financing companies' role in democratizing cosmetic surgery are elitists in denial about their own entrepreneurial activity. He says, "[A] doctor who has made the decision to go into cosmetic surgery has decided to be a businessman" (qtd. in Barry 1998). The president of another new company, Unicorn Financial Services, adds, "Elective procedures have become a consumer product, and consumerism necessitates an ability to finance" (qtd. in Barry 1998).

The Seduction of Commercialism

Letters to the editor and editorials appearing in medical publications provide evidence that not all practitioners are in denial about the entrepreneurial nature of their cosmetic work and its potential for dishonesty, greed, deception, and fraud (e.g., Reddick 1991). Nor are all oblivious to the ethical dilemmas of soliciting patients for elective surgery that can enhance their appearance and quality of life in the best cases but that may endanger their health and even their lives in the worst cases. Not only do some practitioners, mainly board-certified plastic surgeons, recognize the problems that come with commercial medicine, they rail against them, as quotations in this and previous chapters demonstrate. Nevertheless, most have been seduced by the powerful force of commercialism.

The clearest example of this seduction can be seen in the changing activities of the ASPRS. The society understood that opening the legal door to advertising would intensify competition from other types of physicians, given the unrestricted nature of medical licensure. Failing to stop the FTC from applying antitrust law to the learned profession of medicine in 1975, leaders turned to Congress, seeking a legislated exemption from the law or at least restrictions on advertising. Failing to gain any relief at the federal level, they turned to state legislators, who had the power under the states' rights doctrine to provide them some protection by regulating the content of advertising. To date all these efforts have failed to restrict advertising by the ASPRS's competitors as long as it is not false or misleading.

With each successive failure to reestablish regulatory controls over patient solicitation, the ASPRS increased its own marketing efforts on behalf of members. These efforts multiplied after 1975 when the specialty felt increasingly threatened by competition from other specialists who became free to solicit patients. Chapter 4 reveals how the ASPRS stepped up its public relations efforts to "educate" the public about how to choose a qualified physician for cosmetic surgery. The society had to walk a tightrope between the traditional ban against patient solicitation—the ban that it was trying to defend in the political arena—and the economic realities members faced from increased competition for patients. It enlarged its public relations activities again in 1981 to include production of some soft-sell marketing materials for members to use: brochures, patient newsletters, consumer guidebooks, and visual aids. The society also established a telephone referral service and vigorously promoted it in press releases and media interviews. Trying to increase referrals, the society initiated a national advertising campaign in 1985. This campaign focused on defining the ASPRS. It was abandoned when members complained that it did not generate enough new patients to justify the cost. These members wanted the society to focus on increasing consumer demand. Trying to respond to the expressed interests of the majority of members, over the objections of the minority, the society began sponsoring seminars on marketing for members, seminars that included advice on physician advertising, the commercial activity that the society had tried to contain for almost a decade. Despite its battle to assert professional prerogatives over commercial advertising, the marketplace asserted its economic power over the professional specialty and transformed the ASPRS into a commercial trade association. How commercial the society had become was evident in its 1997 advertising campaign aimed at what economists call "supplier-induced demand." The thesis of supplier-induced demand is that physicians can use their culturally recognized superior knowledge to influence demand. Chapter 7 examines the evidence of this phenomenon in women's magazines.

7

Managing the Media Message

Cosmetic Surgery in Women's Magazines

Previous chapters provide evidence that physicians regard women's magazines as one of the most important sources of the public's ideas about cosmetic surgery. Survey data support this belief (Nowak and Washburn 1998). The first major battle in the intraprofessional turf war was caused by an article that appeared in *Harper's Bazaar*. The American Society of Plastic and Reconstructive Surgeons' recently initiated national advertising campaign relied heavily on women's magazines. Public relations efforts by this organization and the others involved with cosmetic surgery, more often than not, target women's magazines. These specialty organizations work aggressively to influence the content of articles and other editorial copy. They pressure writers to include their referral numbers and, more recently, Internet sites. They want more than only a complimentary promotion. They want to manage the media message about cosmetic surgery to promote public demand for their services.

This chapter examines how women's magazines participate in the cultural construction of appearance as a medical problem. While advertising also influences ideology, the messages are usually more limited due to space restrictions. Special advertising supplements would be an exception. Magazine coverage, in contrast, is much less restricted. It is also free and carries an aura of greater legitimacy. Consumer surveys have shown that people prefer media reports to ads as sources of information. This is why the American Society of Plastic and

Reconstructive Surgeons (ASPRS) until recently spent more on public relations than advertising (*Plastic Surgery News* 1989d). Individual physicians continue to turn to public relations services either as a substitute or supplement to advertising campaigns. Typically, they pay monthly retainers of fifteen hundred dollars to firms in the Midwest and to small firms elsewhere. Monthly fees to larger firms on the East or West Coasts can reach six thousand dollars (Glabman 1998). Physicians recognize that public relations are an important part of marketing an elective medical procedure such as cosmetic surgery.

Articles about cosmetic surgery in women's magazines provide readers an opportunity to learn physicians' ideology about the problematic nature of body parts that fall short of the cultural ideal. They instruct readers about the medical interventions available to alter their appearances, who is an appropriate patient, and what are realistic expectations about the surgical experience and outcomes. They also provide a forum for physicians to advance their position in the turf war. This chapter begins with a brief overview of the history of women's magazines and the methods used to examine the content of articles about cosmetic surgery. A discussion of the eight major themes found in cosmetic surgery articles follows. The chapter concludes with a separate discussion of the role of women's magazines in the breast implant crisis of the early 1990s.

Women's Magazines

Unlike magazines targeted at men, women's magazines have survived and multiplied by providing instruction about gender-specific roles, responsibilities, and self-improvement. They began in the early nineteenth century, proselytizing the virtues of piety, purity, submissiveness, and domesticity required for "True Womanhood" (Welter 1973, 211–220). Later, as industrialization reduced the cost of cloth, pattern companies launched fashion magazines. Other new magazines found a niche with a format of short stories, nonfiction, craft projects, and advice about child care and housekeeping. Most of the pattern magazines also expanded to include these same topics (Endres 1995). Subsequently, women's magazines assumed the task of advising readers how to use the continual stream of new domestic appliances, processed food, and cleaning products spun off by industrialization (Fox 1990).

This "service" formula was highly successful. By the early 1980s the dominant "Seven Sisters" (*Ladies' Home Journal, Good Housekeep-*

ing, *McCall's*, *Redbook*, *Better Homes and Gardens*, *Family Circle*, and *Woman's Day*) had a combined circulation of 45 million (Magazine Industry Marketplace 1982). The glossy high-fashion *Vogue* and *Harper's Bazaar*, along with *Glamour*, *Mademoiselle*, *Cosmopolitan*, *New Woman*, *Self*, *Seventeen*, *Teen*, and *Essence* added another 13 million. The success of these magazines ultimately undermined their individual circulations. Publishers aggressively pursued a segment of this lucrative market with new titles ranging from *Sassy* and *YM*, through *Elle*, *Allure*, and *Playgirl*, to *Mirabella* and the supposedly alternative *Ms.*, *Working Woman*, and *Modern Woman*, among others. Nevertheless, the combined circulation of titles aimed at a wide female audience fell to 56 million in 1995 (*National Directory of Magazines* 1995).

Actual readership is higher than circulation indicates because many issues are read by more than one person. More adults read a women's magazine than any other magazine except *TV Guide* and *Reader's Digest* (Simmons Market Research Bureau 1994). Although not all readers of women's magazines are women, these magazines penetrate their target audience to a remarkable extent. For example, one in five adult women read *Better Homes and Gardens* and almost as many read *Good Housekeeping* and *Family Circle*. Readership is higher among white women, women twenty-five and over, and those with at least some college education.

No matter what the targeted age group, race, ethnicity, or socioeconomic level, beauty products and information now command more space than homemaking in most women's magazines. The coverage is particularly intense in those targeted at adolescent girls and young women (Peirce 1990). This change reflects both a response to increased reader interest in physical appearance and beauty product advertisers' demands for a "supportive editorial atmosphere" and "complimentary copy" in exchange for their advertising revenue (Henry 1972; Steinem 1990).

Readers are told how to style their hair, make up their faces, manicure their nails, and dress their bodies to more closely approximate the prevailing ideal. But, the advice does not stop there. Women's magazines offer instruction in how to remake the body itself to meet the prevailing youthful, thin-but-bosomy standard of beauty. Virtually every issue of every major women's magazine in the United States contained instructions on dieting or exercise by the 1980s, and new magazines such as *Pretty Body*, *Shape*, *Weight Watchers*, and *Slimmer* tried to capitalize on the trend (Barber 1982).

Diet and exercise were far less frequently covered before 1970. *Reader's Guide to Periodical Literature* lists only 197 articles on these topics in women's magazines in the 1950s and 230 in the 1960s, compared to 698 in the 1970s. Moreover, articles on cosmetic surgery, a topic rarely covered until the 1980s, are increasingly common. Throughout the 1960s only 15 articles about cosmetic surgery were published in women's magazines indexed by *Reader's Guide* By the 1970s the number increased to 55; it exploded to 107 in the 1980s and kept up the pace with 66 listed from 1990 through 1995. The actual number of such articles is even greater since *Reader's Guide* does not index two of the Seven Sisters, the two that originated as bimonthly "supermarket" magazines, *Women's Day* and *Family Circle*. Nor does *Reader's Guide* index the body-focused *Cosmopolitan* or most of the new diet, fitness, and beauty magazines with comparatively small circulations.

Women's magazines are dismissed by journalists as advertising catalogs and criticized by feminists for not offering positive role models and discussions of social issues to rally women around an agenda for social change (Ferguson 1983; Keller 1994; McCracken 1993; Ruggiero and Weston 1985; Tuchman et al. 1978). Few have considered how women's magazines contribute to the social construction of ideas about health and illness, despite an abundance of health-related coverage. A few exceptions examine what women's magazines tell readers about some specific health issues. For example, women's magazines consistently tell readers that pregnant women over thirty-five are at higher risk and need to have a prenatal diagnosis (Beaulieu and Lippman 1995). Along with other popular magazines, they portray menopause as a "disease" (Mitteness 1983), present toxic shock as a greater risk than it is (Singer and Endreny 1987), and depict premenstrual women as sick and in need of medical, nutritional, psychological, or behavioral therapy (Chrisler and Levy 1990). Discussions of exposure to harmful drugs or pollutants in pregnancy often contain misleading, alarming, and scientifically unsupported information (Gunderson-Warner et al. 1990).

In general women's magazines pay little attention to the most prevalent women's health problems. Although lung cancer surpassed breast cancer as the most deadly cancer among women in the 1980s, six major women's magazines had nothing to say about this alarming development and had virtually nothing to say about any health hazards from smoking (Kessler 1989). Fear of losing tobacco advertising revenue or, in the case of *Good Housekeeping*, which accepts no tobacco advertisements, fear of losing advertising from the food subsidiaries of tobacco companies may well account for why health editors rank lung cancer second to last in terms of reader interest. The only health problem ranked lower is heart disease, the most common cause of death among women. It also is linked to smoking.

Instead of focusing on the most common health problems of women, articles with the appearance-related health themes of dieting, exercise, and nutrition appear twice as frequently in women's magazines, as the second most often covered health issue (Weston and Ruggiero 1985). Together with articles on cosmetic surgery, they constitute one-third of the articles on health issues. Similarly, women's magazines carry almost seven times more over-the-counter drug advertisements than men's magazines, the majority of which are for beauty aids (Vener and Krupka 1986). Women's magazines are, therefore, a significant cultural source of ideas about appearance as a medical problem.

Women's magazines are by no means the only media source amplifying and shaping ideology about cosmetic surgery. American news and business magazines indexed in *Reader's Guide* published 51 articles on cosmetic surgery from 1980 through 1995; however, 37 of these focus on the Food and Drug Administration's (FDA) actions against breast implants and lawsuits against manufacturers. Far more coverage, typically of a positive nature, is provided by newspapers, local magazines, radio, and television. Nevertheless, the intense focus on appearance and long tradition of instruction in self-improvement in women's magazines make their articles about cosmetic surgery particularly powerful. Unlike American news and business magazines, their message is delivered in the context of heightened attention to the importance of appearance. Unlike newspapers, local magazines, and radio, their market is national. Unlike television, their content is more readily accessible for analysis.

Methodology

Reader's Guide to Periodical Literature indexes the content of periodicals by topic. Cosmetic surgery entries are listed under "Surgery, plastic," "Liposuction," and "Breast implants." *Reader's Guide* only indexes articles, a policy that excludes brief discussions of cosmetic surgery in the ubiquitous, composite medical-and-beauty-advice columns and letters to the editor in women's magazines.

Moreover, *Reader's Guide* does not index *Women's Day* and *Family Circle* or new magazines with small circulations. As a result, the 173 articles listed in women's magazines from 1980 through 1995 constitute a large sample of the cosmetic surgery articles in them, rather than the full set of such articles. Two published in *Sassy* were not available for coding, yielding 171 articles for analysis. In spite of these limitations, this set of articles encompasses the large bulk of the discussion of cosmetic surgery in women's magazines available to readers over the sixteen-year period.

The articles were read numerous times to identify common themes and characteristics that were then used to code their content. The aim was to describe the content of the articles as fully as possible. Although much of the thematic content echoes the themes of the ASPRS's Public Education Program, begun in 1977 and expanded in 1982, the content analysis of the articles was completed before the author was aware of this program.

Types of Cosmetic Surgery Articles

Many of the 171 articles discuss more than one surgical procedure. Procedures often are grouped according to their common aesthetic goal, such as changing the profile by modifying the shape of the nose, chin, cheekbones, and ears or reducing the outward signs of aging with eye, brow, and facelifts or with skin treatments. Because some procedures are frequently done at the same time, each article is classified by whether it discusses at least one of the procedures in each broad category (see table 7.1). For example, an article about nose modification, ear pinning, chin extension, and thigh liposuction, is coded only once under the "profile" category and once under the "body contour" category. Chemical peels, dermabrasions, and fat or collagen injections are separated from eye lifts and facelifts because the latter two can involve altering musculature and bone structure while the former only involve skin. Breast reduction is distinguished from augmentation because most physicians and patients argue that the primary motivation for the former is functional, not cosmetic. Breast reductions are included, nonetheless, because there is still debate over the "need" for this elective surgery.

A few cosmetic procedures occur too rarely to code as a separate category. These include a short 1993 *Ladies' Home Journal* article on penile augmentation, a 1994 *Ms.* article lambasting *First for Women* for an article promoting cosmetic genital surgery for women, and two

---

Table 7.1 Cosmetic Surgery Articles in Women's Magazines, 1980–1995

	N	PROFILE	LIFTS	SKIN	BREAST IMPLANT	BREAST REDUC-TION	BODY CON-TOUR
Better Homes & Gardens	5	2	3	3	2	2	4
Essence	2	1			1		
Glamour	16	9	4	1	10	5	5
Good Housekeeping	14	5	5	3	7	6	5
Harper's Bazaar	29	11	22	10	7	4	10
Ladies Home Journal	8	2	4	2	3		2
Lears	1		1				
Mademoiselle	13	7	3	2	11	6	5
McCalls	10	6	6	3	6	3	5
Ms.	7		1		3	1	
Redbook	7	2	3	2	4	1	1
Seventeen	5	4	1	1	2	2	1
Teen	4	4			2	2	2
Vogue	42	8	19	8	9	3	12
Women's Sports & Fitness	3					2	1
Working Mother	1						1
Working Woman	4	1	2	1	2	1	1
Total N	171	62	74	36	69	38	54
% *	100	36	43	21	40	22	31

* The percents do not add to 100 because of articles that discussed more than one type of surgery.

Vogue articles on lip augmentation in 1989 and 1995. Lip augmentation is mentioned briefly in several other articles. Earlobe trimming and scalp reduction are each mentioned once in articles focusing on other procedures.

Three formats dominate. The most common is the instructional guide or update that promises to answer readers' questions about the latest methods and new trends. Nearly two-fifths of the articles fall into this category. These usually provide an overview of the clinical aspects of one or more procedures and costs, along with a typically cursory mention of potential risks and, sometimes, a discussion of how to determine whether you are a good candidate and/or how to choose a physician. Another one-fifth are autobiographical accounts that also mention the motivation for considering cosmetic surgery. These have become increasingly common; nineteen are indexed from 1990 through 1995, compared to fourteen in the 1980s. The third format, also encompassing about one-fifth of the articles, is much like the first except the discussions of procedures are personalized with a description, often accompanied by quotes, of the experience of at least one former patient.

Both the autobiographical articles and those that include the experiences of real patients give readers the opportunity to identify with someone else's discontent about some aspect of her body and consider her solution. Some titles encourage this identification by asking, "Does Your Face Need a Lift?" "Is Liposuction Right for You?" "Breast Reduction Surgery: For You?" or, when multiple procedures are reviewed, "Cosmetic Surgery: Would It Work for You?" "Cosmetic Surgery: Yes or No?" and "Will Changing Your Looks Change Your Life?" Others try to catch the readers' attention with clever titles like "A Stitch in Time," "Eye-Opener," "Waist Not," "Fast Curves," "Getting It Off My Chest," and "Future Perfect." Some of these also have a sidebar or subsection inviting readers to consider whether they should undergo cosmetic surgery.

About one-fifth of the articles do not fit in any of these formats. About half of these are about the breast implant controversy. They are discussed in a separate section. The rest range widely from articles on post-operative care and makeup, video imaging, and cosmetic surgery in the Soviet Union to the results of surveys about cosmetic surgery and two "best" lists of practitioners.

Anti-aging eye, brow, and facelifts are the most frequently reviewed cosmetic operations (see table 7.1). *Vogue* and *Harper's Bazaar* average more than one article a year. Articles on breast implants are a close second, pushed up in rank by a flurry of articles between 1989 and 1993 in response to the Food and Drug Administration's actions to restrict access to silicone-gel implants. Procedures that modify the profile of the head are mentioned next most often, followed by body contouring through tummy tucks, buttock and leg lifts, and liposuction.

Themes
Physicians' Expert Advice

Physicians play a major role as medical experts in the articles. They provide information on the technical nature of the cosmetic procedures and define appearance as a medical problem requiring treatment by an appropriately qualified physician. They also provide information on risks and benefits as well as appropriate motivation and realistic expectations of outcomes and reassure readers that cosmetic surgery is a healthy choice. With the exception of nine autobiographical reports and thirteen others, including seven on the breast implant controversy, a 1989 *Good Housekeeping* reprint of an ASPRS press release on "Who Gets What" cosmetic surgery, and the 1991 *Glamour* survey, all articles include physicians as authorities. Most directly quote or paraphrase physicians and provide their names, cities, affiliations with hospitals, medical schools, centers, institutes, or physicians' organizations, and titles of published books, if any. Ten are written by or with physicians or excerpted from physician-authored cosmetic surgery consumer guidebooks.

The number of physician names appearing in the articles ranges as high as 71 in a list of cosmetic specialists in *Harper's Bazaar*'s 1984 "Who Does What Best." Most articles only cite 1 to 4 physicians. A total of 422 are named in the 171 coded articles in addition to the 71 on the *Harper's Bazaar* list and another 27 on a similar 1981 *Good Housekeeping* list. Some names reappear in numerous articles, others in several, while still others are mentioned only once during the sixteen years of the sample.

All the physicians on the two "best" lists are referred to as plastic surgeons, as are 59 percent of the other 422 mentioned in the articles. Another 8 percent of the 422 physicians are labeled as dermatologists, 5 percent as otolaryngologists, or members of the American Academy of Facial Plastic and Reconstructive Surgery, and 4 percent as simply cosmetic surgeons. About half of the remainder are identified as some other specialist, such as pathologist, immunologist, and rheumatologist, most of whom appear in articles about breast implant safety after 1988, or psychiatrist and surgeon in other articles. The rest are not identified by specialty, even though the text implies that they are experts in cosmetic surgery. Only 30 are women, including 5 in a 1993 *Harper's Bazaar* article deploring the dearth of women physicians offering cosmetic surgery and 6 who are identified as psychiatrists, radiologists, and immunologists.

Medicalization of Appearance

The inclusion of physicians as authorities in the articles contributes to the medicalization of appearance as does the increased number of cosmetic surgery articles. The increased coverage of cosmetic surgery both reflects and contributes to readers' interest in medical procedures to enhance appearance. A 1991 *Glamour* article reports that nearly three-quarters of readers who responded to a survey in a previous issue say that they think the boom in cosmetic surgery is "fine—people should do whatever they feel is necessary to improve their looks." Perhaps more telling, 29 percent of the respondents say they already had cosmetic surgery, 33 percent expect to within the next five to ten years, and another 9 percent say they may when they are much older. Liposuction, breast enlargement, and nose modifications are the procedures most often contemplated by those thinking about cosmetic surgery. Although such voluntary responses are far from representative of all readers they provide editors with support for the expanded coverage of cosmetic surgery. The more articles on cosmetic surgery that women's magazines publish, the more opportunities physicians have to convey their views to the public.

Cosmetic surgery's obvious attraction is its potential to modify appearance to more closely approximate the current ideal. The articles remind readers, "Like it or not, no one can dispute this fact: In this image-conscious world of ours, looks count," as a 1988 *Teen* article says. Some go further and link cosmetic surgery to a moral endeavor. For example, a 1988 *Mademoiselle* article quotes a physician who claims that "youthful beauty, in our culture, is equivalent to good and ugliness to bad." A psychiatrist in this same article suggests, "Patients may unconsciously think of it as baptism by immersion—you go in with your sins around your neck and come up out of the water reborn." A previous 1980 article by two physicians in this magazine argues that even a "relatively minor imperfection, evident to no one but ourselves" cannot be tolerated: "We reject emphatically the fatalistic assumption that there is virtue in tolerating what we perceive to be imperfect."

Vogue's 1995 "Surgical Sculpture" claims, "Thanks to new techniques, cosmetic surgeons say they have become artists, able to shape flesh as finely as Michelangelo crafted marble." The article's conclusion captures the technology-driven medicalization-of-appearance theme that dominates most cosmetic surgery articles:

> Even in the heady world of cosmetic surgery, there are some things money can't buy—not yet, anyway. Surgeons haven't come up with a foolproof way of smoothing out cellulite, for instance. And while breasts can be augmented, there's no good way to build up the buttocks or add girth to calves.
>
> New techniques are certain to come along. Each year "breakthroughs" in cosmetic surgery hit the headlines. . . .
>
> It is also true, of course, that careful diet and regular exercise can't do everything. . . . Body shape, to a significant de-

gree, is inherited. Then, too, there are the ravages of time. Skin sags. Shapes shift. . . . Exercise can slow the inevitable, but it may not be enough. Where regular exercise and a sensible diet leave off, cosmetic surgeons are fond of saying, liposuction begins.

How far we're willing to go down the path toward perfection is something we must decide for ourselves.

According to the articles, the new techniques are an ever evolving array of operations to modify the skin, facial architecture, and body silhouette as well as refresh and rejuvenate aging women.

Surgeons quoted in some articles note that the goal is "now aimed not so much at restoring 'lost youth,' but at giving a woman of any age a more healthful, vital look," or "a chance to improve upon what nature gave them." The healthful, vital, attractive standard projected in the articles consists of smooth, flawless skin, "open" eyes, prominent cheek bones, narrow, straight noses, full lips, chiseled chins, taut jaws and necks, inconspicuous ears, voluptuous breasts, flat stomachs, slim hips and thighs, tight buttocks, and trim knees and ankles. All, readers learn, are "accessible to anyone with a few thousand dollars to spare" for surgery. As *Mademoiselle* announces succinctly in 1988, "Anatomy is no longer destiny," nor is the physical appearance of senescence inevitable. "The technology is fantastic. If one has the resources, there's no reason to look unhandsome at age 80," according to a physician quoted in a 1991 *Better Homes and Gardens*.

Articles frequently refer to cosmetic surgery as a cure for genetic "deformities," even though the attributes labeled as deformities fall well within the normal range of physical variation or age-related changes. For example, liposuction is referred to as a way to cure the contour deformities due to heredity. Nose, chin, and ear modifications and breast augmentation and reduction are similarly presented as treatments for genetic deformities, while facelifts and eye lifts are touted as cures for a "genetic predisposition to wrinkling" and "under eye bags."

Tummy tucks, breast lifts, and thigh and buttocks reductions, in contrast, are presented as techniques to repair the "damage" done by pregnancy and weight gain and loss. Sun exposure and smoking are blamed for skin damage that results in premature aging. Aging that, readers are told, can be rolled back with lifts and either chemical or laser peels. Peels also are promoted to erase the damage from acne and broken blood vessels.

Some articles link cosmetic surgery with treatment of other pathological conditions besides genetic deformities and damage from aging and environmental impacts and note additional physical benefits beyond appearance. Breast reduction, for example, is presented at least partly as a treatment for health problems. Articles suggest it will cure neck and back pain, premenstrual tenderness, shoulder ache, nerve injury, bleeding and scarring from the pressure of bra straps, and rashes and infections caused by heavy breasts rubbing against underlying skin. Several, like a 1985 *Glamour* article, note that physicians say, "We do not regard this as a cosmetic procedure [and] . . . More and more insurance companies realize this." Similarly, some discussions suggest that breathing problems can be cured by rhinoplasty and vision can be enhanced by eye lifts. A 1987 *Harper's Bazaar* article additionally claims that eye lifts can improve "the eye's drainage system and the muscles' ability to blink." The articles also inform readers that insurance companies will pay for these operations if a physician diagnoses a functional problem.

The use of phenol peels is reported to have more than temporary cosmetic benefits in three articles in *Harper's Bazaar* and one in *Vogue* in the 1980s. These articles promise that the collagen connective tissue is altered by the chemical burn and the regenerated skin does not wrinkle as easily. A 1985 *Vogue* article says that peels can remove precancerous lesions before they are visible to the naked eye, a preventive medical intervention. Another 1984 *Vogue* article argues that the problem for some women "is not wrinkles or sagging skin but a sunken look caused by actual shrinkage in the underlying bone structure . . . [due to] osteoporosis." Bone grafts are advocated to rebuild this facial structure. Other articles in the 1990s suggest that the sunken look can be ameliorated by repositioning the falling malar fat pads in the risky, nerve-dense, upper cheek area.

A few articles in the early 1980s promote earlier eye lifts and facelifts as prevention against wrinkles and sagging. A past president of the American Society for Aesthetic Plastic Surgery tells readers, "The younger you are at the initial one, the better they tend to hold. . . . If a woman begins having rejuvenating procedures in her thirties or forties, she'll stay ahead of the aging process more effectively than if she waits until her sixties." Several articles in the late 1980s dispute the benefits of preventive lifts, but not the value of multiple procedures over time. They assure readers that, although the effects are temporary, the operations can be repeated as needed. Examples are given of women who have a "lifetime plan" to "reverse the aging clock" and "maintain [their] 'look.'"

In spite of some debate over preventive lifts in the 1980s, only one of the women undergoing some kind of rejuvenating lift in the 1990s articles is over fifty. She is interviewed in a 1994 *Working Woman* story that discusses age discrimination and how "cosmetic surgery is being marketed as a way to give your career a lift along with your face." The other women mentioned range in age from thirty-five to fifty. Not only do the ages of former patients encourage readers to consider lifts in their thirties and forties, many of the articles in the 1990s explicitly advise readers to have lifts at young ages. For example, a "When to Start" sidebar in a 1990 *Harper's Bazaar* tells readers that some women need eye lifts in their mid to late thirties and a brow lift by their late thirties or early forties. The article's warning that facelifts "should not be deferred too long" because those done before age fifty-five hold up better echoes those published in the early 1980s.

The most extreme examples of cosmetic surgery as preventive medicine appear in *Vogue*'s 1995 "Surgery before 30." The thirty-two-year-old male author reports with some incredulity that "people in their late 20s are having face-lifts . . . to mitigate the earliest signs of aging." He claims that several procedures already are widespread among young models and actresses in their late twenties who want to look like teenagers. These same procedures are being sought by at least some other young women who want, as one told him, a "more chiseled look, much more of a modeled look." These procedures include laser peels, the removal of the buccal fat pad from cheeks, eye lifts, mini facelifts that pull the eyes toward the temples, and lip augmentations. A surgeon interviewed about the trend declares, "I love working with young people! The skin is just in such good shape. It bounces right back. . . . There is a better end result." She further suggests, "You never physically have to go through looking middle-aged." A second surgeon adds, "If you do these relatively small procedures earlier, you have less to do later."

How to Choose Dr. Right

As discussed in previous chapters, the ASPRS has engaged in an extensive marketing campaign to sell the public on the idea that only board-certified plastic surgeons are qualified to do cosmetic surgery. Although nonplastic surgeons have successfully defended their legal right to do cosmetic surgery under the American

Medical Association (AMA) and Federal Trade Commission (FTC) policies, they have not been as successful in conveying their position to the public. How to choose a physician for cosmetic surgery is one of the most prevalent themes in the women's magazine articles. In the vast majority of these articles, the readers are told to find a board-certified plastic surgeon. How to choose Dr. Right is the primary theme of six articles, and a secondary theme in almost 40 percent of the others. Articles without this theme include many of the personal stories, twenty-four on the breast implant controversy and the FDA's actions, and those on atypical topics such as cosmetic surgery resorts, video imaging, post-surgical use of cosmetics, and trends in male cosmetic surgery.

Providing how-to instruction is consistent with the traditional role of women's magazines and is present in articles on other health topics, such as nutrition, exercise, first aid, and disease prevention. However, telling readers how to choose among physicians for medical care, suggesting that some physicians are unqualified to provide the kinds of medical care they offer, and providing free advertising for referral services operated by speciality associations are highly unusual messages in women's magazines, other than in their articles about cosmetic surgery. These messages echo the infamous 1960 *Harper's Bazaar* article that led to the hostility between plastic surgeons and otolaryngologists. They also are the central themes of the Public Education Program adopted by the ASPRS's Board of Directors in 1982 and promoted by its public relations efforts (Hugo 1982). A few articles also reflect the public relations responses of competing speciality associations, but, overwhelmingly, the views of the ASPRS dominate the articles in women's magazines.

The discussion of how to choose a physician is often set off with a subtitle like "Selecting a Surgeon" or "Buyer Beware" or highlighted in a sidebar, such as "Picking a Surgeon" in *Better Homes and Gardens'* 1987 "Cosmetic Surgery Today" or "If You're Going to Do It, at Least Get a Good Doctor" in *Mademoiselle's* 1994 "4 True Tales of Plastic Surgery." The unusually skeptical tone of the last example reflects the poor outcomes of two tales—one about a woman who was hospitalized twenty-three times after an implant ruptured in a car accident and the other about a woman whose nose had to be repaired after a botched first operation. Emphasizing the importance of careful selection, this woman tells readers that she went to the "best" doctor at the "best" place, the nationally renowned Mayo Clinic, for her second operation.

Almost all articles that discuss how to choose a physician, as well as a few others, tell readers to see a board-certified plastic surgeon. About one-fourth of those that discuss physician selection, as well as four others, suggest a board-certified facial plastic surgeon, dermatologist, or ophthalmologist as an option in addition to, or instead of, a board-certified plastic surgeon. Only five suggest a board-certified cosmetic surgeon. More warn against choosing self-described cosmetic surgeons, even if they are members of the American Academy of Cosmetic Surgery. Several articles quote plastic surgeons who question the screening criteria of this competing organization, whose certification, they warn readers, is not recognized by the American Board of Medical Specialties, a distinction that is not always clearly explained.

Other board-certified plastic surgeons try to differentiate themselves from physicians such as otolaryngologists, whose board-certification is recognized by the American Board of Medical Specialities, by emphasizing plastic surgeons' extensive training in reconstructive work. Many more talk generally about the need for careful selection of a physician because unnamed "unqualified" practitioners who are not adequately trained in plastic and reconstructive techniques can offer cosmetic surgery. For example, a 1980 *Seventeen* article tells readers that their expert consultants warn that finding a good cosmetic surgeon "can be confusing, since several surgical specialty groups 'certify' doctors, but not all such certifications are trustworthy. What's more, any MD can legally perform plastic surgery." Readers are told about the qualifications of ASPRS members and cautioned by one to "be sure you are not dealing with a doctor who calls himself a plastic surgeon just because he does some plastic surgery." This message is repeated throughout the sixteen years, often with dire warnings. For example, a 1991 *Teen* article tells readers that they need a physician who has "passed the boards (tests) of the American Board of Plastic Surgery, Inc." because "the right surgeon can (sometimes literally) make or break your face."

The extensive attention given to choosing a physician for cosmetic surgery reflects the bitter intraprofessional turf battle between board-certified plastic surgeons and other physicians who engage in cosmetic surgery. Seven articles explicitly tell readers about this turf battle. Unlike the vast majority of articles that discuss how to select a physician, most of these seven advise that there is disagreement between physician groups over who is best qualified to do particular cosmetic procedures and suggest that readers can choose depending on a physician's training and experience. For example, *Vogue*'s 1989 "Images: Reshaping" accuses the physicians' groups of acting like the Hatfields and McCoys: "Each insists that it is the more legitimate enterprise. It's more than likely that both associations are made up of good surgeons and a few lemons."

Like the 1989 congressional hearings on cosmetic surgery, the articles on the turf battle express concern about the proliferation of cosmetic surgery advertising and warn readers against choosing a physician based on advertising hype. This message appears in a few other articles as well. For example, a 1988 *Vogue* cautions readers that unqualified physicians are "using advertising techniques that have dangerously and unrealistically, altered our perception of cosmetic surgery as now being safe, simple, predictable." Rather than elaborating on possible health complications and the social, economic, and psychological pressures on women to look attractive, the article discusses how to find "Dr. Right," who can safely provide the best aesthetic result with the least risk.

Readers are advised to consult friends, family physicians, local medical directories, and referral services sponsored by physicians' speciality associations. More than half of the articles provide addresses or telephone numbers for one of these referral services. The success of the board-certified plastic surgeons' Public Education Campaign is readily apparent; 46 percent of the 171 articles mention the ASPRS's referral service, compared to 12 percent that mention the otolaryngologists' American Academy of Facial Plastic and Reconstructive Surgery and only 4 percent that mention the American Academy of Cosmetic Surgery. The few articles suggesting that readers contact the latter for referrals were mostly published in 1988 and 1989 in response to press releases issued by this new organization. The telephone number for this association's referral service, last mentioned in a 1991 *Essence* article, was no longer in service by 1996.

In addition to establishing a prospective physician's professional credentials, readers are advised to ask about amount of experience, proportion of practice devoted to the desired procedure, whether he or she has privileges to do the procedure in a hospital in the proximity of peers, and whether an ambulatory site is equipped with resuscitation equipment and accredited. These questions are standard ASPRS recommendations. Some additionally suggest asking to see a physician's before-and-after photographs. Others discount the value of photographs or suggest talking with former patients. Readers are cautioned against physicians who promise radical changes, avoid discussing possible complications, or encourage additional procedures not related to the problem presented by the patient. The right doctor, a 1991 *Teen* article reminds readers, "will advise you to do what's in your best interests, not to supplement his income."

Risks

The tone of most articles is relentlessly positive and sometimes lighthearted. A few examples include *Ladies' Home Journal*'s "I'm in Love With My New Face," *Good Housekeeping*'s "The Happiest Decision I Ever Made," *McCall*'s "Cosmetic Surgery for Real Women," and *Women's Sports and Fitness*'s "One Woman's Liberation." The major exceptions are twenty-four articles exclusively on breast implants, published after the FDA began a review of implants in 1988. These will be discussed separately.

Only eight other articles emphasize the risks of a cosmetic operation more than the benefits. One is *Mademoiselle*'s "4 True Tales of Plastic Surgery," in which two tales are negative: a shocking story on breast implants and a subsequently corrected nose bob that left a patient temporarily disfigured. Another is *Glamour*'s 1988 "The Cosmetic Surgery Hoax," which focuses on health risks and poor aesthetic outcomes as well as the turf battle over cosmetic surgery. Despite only presenting negative examples of cosmetic surgery, it concludes, "Not all cosmetic surgery turns out badly. Most of it turns out pretty much as planned." Moreover, it contains a sidebar, "How to Check up on a Cosmetic Surgeon," which implies that serious problems can be avoided if readers select their physicians carefully.

The other articles in which the presentation of risks overshadows benefits focus on one kind of surgery. These include two on facelifts in the same 1981 *Harper's Bazaar*, one on liposuction in a 1989 *Vogue*, a personal account in a 1991 *Good Housekeeping* of a woman left with pain, a distorted face, and nerve damage from silicone injections to build up her cheekbones, and the 1994 *Ms.* article criticizing *First for Women* for promoting female genital surgery. The *Ms.* author dismisses the *First for Women* article as a "dreadful piece in a dreadful magazine." But, she also claims that other "smarter" women's magazines "venture onto the same slippery slope" by minimizing the risks in their enthusiastic coverage of cosmetic surgery. She further chastises them for playing on women's insecurities, encouraging women to become self-absorbed, and feeding women's worst obsessions.

Negative articles on facelifts, nose modifications, and liposuction stress the unreliable aesthetic results more than health risks, as do a few generally favorable articles on these and other procedures. For example, 1989 and 1995 *Vogue* articles on lip enlargement and other discussions of collagen, fibril, and fat injections into acne scars and facial creases, although not advising readers against the procedures, stress the temporary duration of change, a matter of two or three months. Many articles on facelifts or eye lifts similarly note that these changes are not permanent, but the duration is measured in years, not months. A few others, including a fairly negative personal report of a facelift in a 1986 *Ms.* and a report on liposuction in a 1993 *Essence*, offer cautionary tales. These articles stress the need to select a qualified physician or express concern about trying to find self-esteem through surgery.

Approximately 35 percent of the articles tell readers nothing about the health risks of cosmetic surgery other than, in some articles, the temporary side effects common to any medical procedure—swelling, discoloration, numbness—and the potential for infection. Another 16 percent say that there is a possibility of other complications without specifying them. The 28 percent of articles that briefly mention specific risks, such as potentially deadly reactions to anesthesia, nerve damage, facial paralysis, vision problems, or blood clots, dismiss them as rare and typically stress the importance of physician selection, as mentioned in a previous section. Only 22 percent discuss health risks in sufficient detail to emphasize cautious consideration of the possibility of physical complications, as well as choice of physician, when thinking about cosmetic surgery. The eight articles judged to emphasize risks more than benefits fall into this last category along with others that provide examples of good outcomes and patients who are happy with their cosmetic surgery.

The frequent link made between physical risks, whether mentioned briefly or in somewhat more detail, and selection of a physician implies that the issue of physical risks is only a facet of the larger issue of physician selection. This view is underscored by the comments of medical experts and further highlighted in a few articles, such as a 1988 *Glamour* article informing readers that some physicians claim that from 5 to 25 percent of their work is repairing aesthetic or medical damage inflicted by less skilled practitioners. Only one article, in the October 1989 *Vogue*, discloses, "Even the best surgeon is only human and does occasionally make mistakes. Things don't quite work out not because he's incompetent but because things don't always go perfectly." Most articles give readers the opposite impression by minimizing the discussion of specific physical risks and emphasizing the importance of physician selection.

Specific aesthetic and health risks are most often mentioned in reports about eye lifts, liposuction, and breast augmentation and reduction and least often mentioned in connection with ear pinning. If readers of women's magazines read all of the articles on eye lifts over the sixteen years, they would learn that the removal of excess fat and skin above or below the eye can result in one eye appearing to be larger or higher than the other and one or both looking sunken or showing an excessive amount of white beneath the iris. Besides these poor aesthetic results and the potential risk of anesthesia shared by all surgery, eye lifts also can result in excessive watering, dry eye, inability to fully close eyes, corneal damage, blurred vision, and, in rare cases, blindness.

Liposuction, the most popular cosmetic operation by the late 1980s, was only introduced in the United States in 1982. It began as a relatively crude procedure in which a cannula attached to a vacuum device was repeatedly thrust into deep body fat. That technique required more physical strength than finesse.

The first information about liposuction in women's magazines, such as *Good Housekeeping*'s 1985 "The Operation That Did What All My Diets Didn't Do!" presents it as the ultimate solution for frustrated dieters who were unable to rid themselves of localized fat on outer thighs and the stomach. Liposuction never is touted as a treatment for obesity. Instead, it is presented as a technique to refine an already fit silhouette. Later articles warn of poor aesthetic results—rippled, dimpled, loose skin—and possible complications—infection, inflammation, muscle and nerve damage, bowel perforation, blood clots, excessive blood and body-fluid loss, and shock. Only four articles, however, acknowledge there have been deaths.

Liposuction articles in the 1990s mention past problems and inform readers about new technological improvements. Less traumatic, smaller cannulas, hand-held syringes, and the new "tumescent technique," readers are told, promise improved outcomes. The latter involves injecting fluid laced with a local anesthesia to separate fat cells from connective tissue and avoids the risks of general anesthesia in some cases. The new, refined instruments can be used on more superficial deposits of fat to make cheekbones more prominent and trim jowls, chin, upper arms, kneecaps, calves, and ankles. Two articles in the mid-1990s announce that physicians can now etch the "washboard" stomach of a bodybuilder using these new techniques. Besides one negative 1989 *Vogue* article, the dominant message, like the messages about other cosmetic procedures, is that the risks are small compared to the benefits for those who have appropriate expectations about the aesthetic outcome of "body sculpting" and pick the right physician.

Breast reduction reports almost always warn readers about the scars and the possible loss of nipple sensation and ability to breast feed. Articles in the 1990s stress techniques to preserve the nipple. Previously, only *Mademoiselle*'s 1986 "Hard Facts about Cosmetic Surgery" warns that women can lose their nipples or that repeat surgery to correct asymmetrical healing is common. The rest stress that the risks are outweighed by the benefits of smaller breasts.

Social and Economic Benefits

Despite some titles that suggest otherwise, none of the articles promises that cosmetic surgery will improve your life. Many explicitly state that it will not solve life's problems, or save a marriage or a job. However, some of these same articles, as well as others, suggest that it could make a difference; they discuss former patients whose lives were transformed or who say simply that they are happier now. Some of these women talk about the misery of being teased for their big breasts, nose, or ears as teenagers, or about their obsession with their fat thighs and ankles or flat chests. *Better Homes and Gardens'* 1993 "The Healing Power of Plastic Surgery: It's More Than Just Skin Deep" offers a good example of the mixed message. The authors say, "Modern medicine may improve your appearance, but it won't solve your other problems," only two paragraphs after quoting a dermatologist who claims, "I've seen patients who were afraid to leave home. . . . When their skin problems were corrected, their lives turned around."

Several articles claim that the benefits sought vary by sex. *Harper's Bazaar*'s 1991 "Youth Lifts" opines that women are driven to cosmetic surgery by "romantic desires . . . wanting to maintain their appeal to husbands or mates," whereas men's "impetus is business-related." Articles in *Working Woman* disagree. The 1988 "Career Woman's Guide to Cosmetic Surgery" says, "Many high-achieving women—even those who previously shunned the concept of cosmetic surgery as frivolous—are beginning to wonder whether a straighter nose, a stronger chin or more youthful-looking eyes could translate into increased dollars and success in the marketplace." Moreover, the article notes that surveys indicate, "many people believe a youthful appearance and physical attractiveness are key ingredients for achieving power and success on the job." Six years later, "Face Value" provides numerous examples of professional women, celebrities, and several well-known feminists who have had cosmetic surgery. The author informs readers about the economic studies that find men and women who are rated below average in attractiveness typically earn less than those rated above average. Although the author warns that the positive changes some patients experience may be secondary effects of enhanced self-confidence, the author also notes that "[i]n an era in which corporations are slashing budgets and laying off older workers," readers need to be concerned about their image.

The message is the same in magazines aimed at a minority audience. An African American surgeon in a 1991 *Essence* article comments, "Society is saying that you cannot be successful if you're not good-looking. Many things are based, and many assumptions are made, on how you look. It's not fair, but it's true." Surgical modification of racially distinctive features, although increasing, remains highly controversial. This article warns that friends may accuse cosmetic patients of racial self-hatred. However, the chief of plastic surgery at Howard tells readers that this pathological motivation is only true for 10 to 20 percent of patients and suggests that they will be better served by a physician who shares their cultural background and understands their desire to soften a prominent feature or beautify themselves, not make themselves less African American.

There is a sexual undertone to many discussions, particularly those about breast implants before the controversy over safety arose. A 1984 *Vogue* points out, "You won't have to wear falsies. You'll probably feel you look better in a bathing suit, as well as naked." A 1986 *Mademoiselle* quotes a cosmetic surgeon who says that all his patients "have lots of fun buying new lingerie" because of the "instant zaftig" he gives them. Even a negative 1980 *Good Housekeeping* article about a mother of three who changed her mind about her implants says that she did so because of men's response to her new body. She says, "The reaction was a teenager's dream come true. Men ran to open doors for me. Sales men tripped over one another to wait on me. My male professors took renewed interest in me." Readers might regard her experience as a positive benefit. Similarly, a 1988 *Mademoiselle* article describes a "top model" who claims, "I got a part on a primetime TV series only two weeks later because of my [implanted] breasts." She also says that she became romantically involved with the star of the show because he thought that she had "the most beautiful breasts God has ever given a woman."

Not all the suggestions that cosmetic surgery will improve a patient's sex life are limited to breast implants. The author of a 1985 *Good Housekeeping* article tells how her weight problems made her feel "so frumpy" that she avoided physical intimacy with her husband. After liposuction she could wear pants three sizes smaller. "More important, I've regained my old self-confidence and a sense of control over the way I look." Her husband was "happier than ever." As several of these examples demonstrate, some of the implied or suggested social and economic benefits are presented as secondary effects of psychological changes.

Mental Health Benefits

Approximately one-third of the articles explicitly claim that the benefits of cosmetic surgery extend beyond physical changes to mental health. Many of these, including a 1985 *Vogue* article, associate the growing demand for cosmetic surgery with the healthy narcissism that led to concern about exercise and diet in the 1980s. Physicians quoted in these articles promote the idea that the physical changes, whether dramatic as with breast implants or subtle as with facelifts, result in a more positive body image, improved self-esteem, self-confidence, and sense of well-being. Some articles suggest additional psychological benefits from particular operations. Breast augmentation is linked to feeling more womanly and being less likely to have sexual difficulties. Breast reduction is touted to relieve the strain of being stared at and treated as a sex object. A Beverly Hills physician generalizes in a 1989 *Vogue*, "Cosmetic surgery is quick and cheap psychotherapy." Former patients are quoted who make the same claims.

The articles make clear that the psychological benefits are not limited to those whose appearance falls far short of the cultural ideal. A 1988 *Glamour* article, for example, claims that "there are few ugly ducklings in the waiting rooms of plastic surgeons. . . . the typical cosmetic surgery patient is a woman of average or above average looks who wants to look even better." Most articles present this desire as an admirable trait. A 1988 *Teen* article discusses how craniofacial surgery "transformed Amy from an average-looking girl into a pretty young lady." Bone grafts from the back of Amy's eighteen-year-old head built up her cheekbones, and her jawbone was shortened by one-quarter of an inch and reattached with plates held by screws. The article notes that Amy "had to think twice—even a few times—before okaying the surgery . . . [which] 'hadn't been performed very much,' says Amy, 'so they couldn't show me before and after pictures.'"

The implication that Amy was hesitant is typical of personal stories of women of all ages. Many speak of pre-operation anxiety and doubts. They say or imply that cosmetic surgery is a difficult decision and that women must be courageous to submit to the knife for beauty. A fifty-two-year-old interior decorator in a 1980 *Ladies' Home Journal* article relates that she agonized over an eye lift and was sure the physician would say she did not need it. Instead, she says, "[He] showed me what a face-lift, as well as an eye operation, would do for me. I was convinced."

In spite of claims about cosmetic surgery's mental health benefits, articles also warn that postoperative depression is common. The interior decorator, like women in other articles, says that after the operation she sobbed and wondered, "Why am I doing this to myself?" and sank into depression when she saw her painful, swollen, discolored face. After ten days in the hospital and another few days at home, "returning to [her] office . . . was a great test of strength." Nevertheless, after a month passed and coworkers complimented her appearance, she felt, "[I] gained five years, not just because of the way I look but also because of the new lift in my step and the renewed self-confidence," and she concluded, "[C]oping with the operation and the aftermath has given me quite a feeling of accomplishment."

Proper Motivation and
Realistic Expectations

Although the social, economic, and psychological benefits of cosmetic surgery are common themes, almost half of the articles, excluding those on the breast implant controversy, say or imply that some seek cosmetic surgery for inappropriate reasons. These articles discuss "right" and "wrong" motivations. Readers are instructed to do it for themselves, not for others. Physicians consistently describe the best candidates as physically healthy individuals with realistic expectations, who are emotionally stable, self-motivated, and not unreasonably concerned about physical imperfections. Such patients are more likely to be satisfied with their outcomes. In spite of numerous statements to the contrary, many of these articles caution that cosmetic surgery will not change a person's social life, solve personal problems, cure depression, or change a personality. Like many articles that discuss mental health benefits, a 1980 *Teen* article claims it will make "you feel better about yourself and your appearance which, in turn boosts your confidence."

Articles aimed at older readers similarly caution that "cosmetic surgery does not cure depression or social anxiety, nor does it convert self-hatred into self-love" and that it "won't reform a wayward husband, rekindle a dormant romance, or salvage a dying marriage." Instead, a physician in a 1980 *McCall's* says that it allows older patients "to reaffirm to themselves and others that they are still youthful and effective. This is especially true after a loss—whether it's of a husband through divorce or death, of children who leave home, of fertility after menopause." The physician elaborates that cosmetic surgery "should be viewed as a facilitator of change rather than a basic change in the individual's personality, behavior or approach to life." Other articles make this same point with examples, such as a widow in her late forties whose facelift stimulated her to take secretarial courses and find a job. *Good Housekeeping* readers in 1981 learn that "her personality took on a sparkle that made her fun to be around. As a result, she now has an active social life."

Few acknowledge that patients either may be unconscious of their real motives for cosmetic surgery or may deliberately dupe their physicians. One exception, a 1988 *Mademoiselle* article, tells of an eighteen-year-old tummy-tuck patient who claimed to be too embarrassed about her stomach after a pregnancy to have a sexual relationship. The physician only discovered her sexual phobia after operating on her when she announced that she still could not have sexual relations because of the surgical scar.

Standards for accepting patients appear to vary. A physician in a 1980 *Seventeen* article claims that psychiatric examinations are not necessary because cosmetic surgery is "basically happy surgery." He tells his young readers, "[T]here's nothing wrong with wanting to improve your looks, as long as you're willing to accept the limitations of an operation." Some, like one in a 1982 *Vogue,* assert, "A history of neurotic conflicts does not, however, necessarily contraindicate having cosmetic surgery. The offending physical feature may in fact be contributing to the patient's emotional distress. Even depressed patients might benefit from surgery." In contrast, others say they turn away patients who are unduly concerned about their features, suffer from Body Dysmorphic Disorder (in which a perceived imperfection is greatly exaggerated), or blame their appearance for all their problems. A physician in a 1982 *Vogue* admits, "In such cases, only close collaboration between patient, plastic surgeon, and psychiatrist should determine when and if surgery is wise."

The rapid growth in cosmetic surgery advertising and public acceptance have led the nonphysician authors of nine articles to express concern that these trends may create "scalpel slaves," women who seek a sense of self-worth and happiness through multiple operations. A 1988 *Mademoiselle* article provides the example of a twenty-four-year-old who had had three nose jobs, a facial peel, cheek implants, and breast augmentation, as well as fat sucked from her buttocks and injected into her lips. Although these articles note that such examples make up only a small minority of patients, they also acknowledge that it is common to have more than one procedure. A 1990 study, mentioned in a 1995 *Working Woman* article, reports that 95 percent of female and 78 percent of male patients are willing to have more cosmetic surgery. In fact, all the former patients interviewed for this feature article planned to have more work done.

The authors of these articles imply that psychotherapy would be more appropriate for patients who repeatedly undergo cosmetic surgery. Their message, however, is mixed with examples of women who are very happy with the results of their multiple surgeries. One is a twenty-four-year-old who received national notoriety as professional playboy Hugh Hefner's girlfriend. Some readers may be more impressed with her achieved celebrity status than with the author's concern that women like her are "cosmetic surgery junkies." Moreover, the author reports that most of the interviewed physicians believe that repeat surgery does not mean a patient is a scalpel slave because everyone is body-conscious. Even a 1988 *Glamour* article that takes a dim view of multiple cosmetic operations concludes that if a woman has "basic self-confidence, changing the one part of her body that bothers her will only enhance her feelings about herself."

Censuring patients who want additional procedures would be difficult for physicians whose livelihood depends on their business. Moreover, repeat surgery is inevitable and treated as normative for those striving to maintain the youthful cultural ideal with facelifts and eye lifts.

Everybody's Doing It

The normative nature of cosmetic surgery is the last of the dominant themes evident in the articles in women's magazines. Readers are reassured that cosmetic surgery is a morally, socially, economically, and psychologically appropriate choice. For example, a 1985 *Vogue* article points out, "the demographics of plastic surgery have shifted: no longer are patients only movie stars or the super-rich; they are also stockbrokers, executive secretaries, lawyers, school teachers, even members of the clergy . . . who want to look better, less tired, refreshed." Overall, 62 percent of the articles explicitly mention how popular cosmetic surgery has become among people like the readers or provide statistics to convey this impression.

The proportion of articles providing specific examples of women who have elected cosmetic surgery has increased from 44 percent in the 1980s to 70 percent from 1990 through 1995, excluding those on the breast implant controversy. Most are middle- and upper-middle-class white females. Only four articles focus on men and only the two *Essence* articles discuss African Americans and Hispanics. Reader identification is further enhanced by mentioning their ages, which mirror those of each magazine's readership.

The desire to surgically alter appearance is treated as normative for teenagers as well. Teen and preteen readers are told, "More and more teens are choosing plastic surgery. That's why *Teen*'s talked with some great gals who've put their faces (and figures) in the hands of plastic surgeons—and couldn't be more pleased with the results." *Seventeen* tells them not only that "there's nothing wrong with wanting to improve your looks," but also, "If [your parents] are unsympathetic (and some are), a teacher, minister or counselor may be able to reopen the discussion."

The examples and statistics serve to normalize the choice of cosmetic surgery and affirm that it is socially acceptable and no longer an option only for the wealthy. The latter message is reinforced with information on the cost of procedures in 51 percent of the articles, other than those on the breast implant controversy. Physicians reassure hesitant readers that the decision to have cosmetic surgery is more likely to be a sign of mental health than of excessive self-absorption. A 1989 *McCall's* article declares that "it isn't even a matter of being vain—it's a matter of having a healthy, forward outlook." In several articles, reluctant patients are treated as deviant by physicians who say they need help to overcome guilt about altering their appearance or spending so much money on themselves.

The Breast Implant Controversy

The content and tone of breast implant discussions changed radically after medical researchers, pathologists, and rheumatologists raised questions about implant deterioration and the potential for carcinogenic effects and autoimmune reactions. Under pressure from a 1990 congressional hearing on the medical problems reported by some women with implants, the FDA reclassified these devices and required manufacturers to submit scientific evidence of their safety in 1991. After discovering there was a lack of reliable scientific information on the safety of breast implants, the government agency called for a moratorium on silicone gel-filled breast implants in 1992.

Prior to 1989, women's magazines promoted breast implants. If an article on breast implants mentioned a potential problem, it was most likely capsular contracture. Capsular contracture occurs when scar tissue forms around an implant, tightens, and makes the breast hard and, in some cases, distorted or painful. The estimated incidence reported in various articles ranges from 15 to 50 percent. Some of these articles suggest that alternative locations for implant placement and alternative implant designs, such as polyurethane foam-coated implants, can reduce the likelihood of the problem. Other risks mentioned, although infrequently, include decreased sensitivity, problems detecting cancerous tumors on mammograms, leakage, immunological reactions, hematomas (a collection of blood around the implant), and infection.

Most reports that mention breast implant risks before 1989 dismiss the risks as minimal. Those that mention them tell readers that they can be reduced with careful choice of a physician and that if they occur, they can be fixed. Readers are informed that physicians can try to break up scar tissue by vigorously squeezing the breasts, although subsequent reports warn this could cause a rupture. Readers also are advised in some articles that scar tissue can be surgically removed and the implant replaced. A few articles, including a 1981 physician-authored *Glamour* report, question whether breast hardness is a true complication. This physician adds that fears of cancer are "groundless" and mammography "is not blocked and, in fact, I am often told by radiologists that it is easier to read and interpret a mammogram after the placement of the implant beneath breast tissue." He provides no evidence to substantiate his claims. Medical experts in other articles, particularly after the late 1980s, contradict his assertions. They instruct readers to tell their mammogram technicians about their

```
┌─────────────────────────────────────────┐
│                                         │
│         ARE YOU A CANDIDATE             │
│         FOR COSMETIC SURGERY            │
│                                         │
│   Do you have a physical feature that really │
│       bothers you?                      │
│   Do you have difficulty breathing through │
│       your nose because of an abnormality? │
│   Do you have difficulty chewing because your │
│       jaws don't fit together properly? │
│   Do you have excessive wrinkling?      │
│   Do you have acne scars?               │
│   Do you have a "turkey gobbler's" neck? │
│   Do frown lines make you look angry all the │
│       time?                             │
│   Do you have such bags around your eyes that │
│       you constantly look tired or dissipated? │
│   Do your ears protrude?                │
│   Are your breasts so small that you have │
│       trouble getting dresses that fit? │
│   Are your breasts so heavy that you have │
│       neck, shoulder, back, and skin    │
│       discomfort?                       │
│   Do you have flabby thighs, abdomen, and/or │
│       buttocks that are out of proportion to the │
│       rest of you?                      │
│   Are you in reasonably good health?    │
│   Can you afford the time and money for a │
│       cosmetic plastic-surgery procedure? │
│                                         │
└─────────────────────────────────────────┘
```

Figure 7.1. Are you a candidate for cosmetic surgery? *From "The Complete Book of Plastic Surgery" by Michael Hogan and Ruth Winter,* Good Housekeeping,*1981.*

implants because special procedures must be used to offset the tendency of implants to obscure breast x-rays.

Most articles published immediately after the 1988 release of a study linking silicone to breast cancer in rats reassure readers, some of whom would be among the then estimated two million American women with implants. Physicians are quoted who challenge the study's findings and assert that there is no evidence of an elevated cancer risk in humans. A 1989 *Mademoiselle* report declares, "[T]he medical community, almost universally, has declared the findings of the rat study to be completely inapplicable to humans."

When FDA scientists at the end of 1990 leaked findings that the exterior of polyurethane foam-covered implants breaks down into known carcinogens, Surgitek, which had acquired the patent from another company only a year before, stopped shipment and issued a press release to reassure women, as did the FDA, the ASPRS, and other physicians' organizations. Physicians' credibility had been damaged. The 1991 articles reflect a more cautious view on the part of journalists about the risks of implants. Nevertheless, most continued to convey to their readers the message that physicians wanted them to hear, although the tone of the articles indicated some skepticism about physicians' honesty on this issue. The May *Mademoiselle* declares, "the jury is still out." The July *Ladies' Home Journal* warns nervous readers with implants that the risk involved in the general anesthesia needed to remove them is greater than the small risk of cancer from them and suggests that other readers considering implants "might want to wait." Others suggest considering saline implants or fat transplants as alternatives.

Taking a more critical position, the August *Glamour* reviews the checkered history of foam-covered implants in a five-page exposé. The exposé claims that there was medical evidence in the mid-1970s that women's tissues grow into the polyurethane foam covers. When the company then making them stopped, one of its salesmen bought the patent and continued production in his garage. To stimulate interest, he gave his implants to surgeons willing to conduct clinical trials and rewarded at least one, for publishing a positive report in 1984, with 3.5 percent of the sale price on every one sold. Increased sales (probably boosted by the unacknowledged flurry of favorable coverage in women's magazines) led to his company's acquisition by another medical-device firm in 1987. That firm quickly sold the business to Surgitek, a subsidiary of Bristol-Myers Squibb, after a 1988 FDA inspection found a general lack of sterile techniques in production. Although the *Glamour* article acknowledged that Surgitek responded expeditiously when evidence of potential carcinogens emerged, the other facts in the article were unlikely to allay readers' fears about this type of implant or reassure them that they could trust what physicians said about implants and, by extension, cosmetic surgery in general.

The backlash expanded when other questions about implants emerged. A few rheumatologists and former patients suggested there was a link between silicone gel and connective-tissue diseases due to autoimmune reactions. The publicity given these concerns and lack of scientific data on safety led the FDA to ask for a voluntary moratorium on all silicone-gel implants in January 1992 over the objections of the ASPRS and other physician groups involved in cosmetic surgery. Women's magazines responded with widespread coverage; fifteen articles about implants are listed in *Reader's Guide* in 1991 and 1992.

Cosmetic surgery practitioners interviewed by journalists continue to reassure readers. For example, a 1991 *Harper's Bazaar* report says physicians believe, "There is essentially no objective, scientifically credible evidence that silicone causes cancer or collagen vascular disease," and it advises against implant removal. Reporters, nonetheless, express their new skepticism in articles with sensational titles like "My Twenty-Year Nightmare," "A Body to Die For," and "If You Have Breast Implants . . . Now What." Some of these discuss women who have had numerous operations to replace ruptured or hardened implants and remove scar tissue or drain blood accumulation, well-established complications rarely mentioned in previous coverage.

Seven of the fifteen articles published in 1991 and 1992 complain that the FDA was negligent for not requiring evidence of implant safety sooner. A pathologist in one article complains, "We've performed an experiment on millions of women with an unproven medical device." Two other articles overtly question whether plastic and other cosmetic surgeons can be trusted to give objective information about the risks of implants. Five others tell readers to seek support and information from the recently established Command Trust Network. Six, including one in 1994, also discuss ongoing court cases or suggest what readers need to do to prepare for a lawsuit. A 1992 *Vogue* article concludes,

> The story of breast implants isn't the simple one it once seemed—not a story of technology triumphant over the limits of the body, but one of wishful thinking, greed, and gullibility. . . . everyone in this morality play has a good reason to subtly skew the plot line. Money is one: there are large sums on all sides of this issue, as much, potentially, for lawyers as plastic surgeons ever brought home. Philosophy is another, the great divide between those who rush to fix every

departure from society's physical ideal and those who are less obsessed, or more puritanical. And of course, there's tactical maneuvering going on: while all the FDA's thunder is justified—belated, but justified—the volume also serves to make up for years of inaction and to put other companies on notice that the agency is getting tougher.

The intense coverage in women's magazines helped create the crisis atmosphere that led to one of the most expensive class-action lawsuits in American history. There was little follow-up; only six articles on breast implants are listed in the next three years. One in 1993 suggests that readers consider saline implants or other alternatives such as fat transplants. Only seven articles over the sixteen years question the cultural influences that pressure women to equate femininity and personal value with large breasts. And only one points to the role that the media play in supporting medical solutions to appearance concerns. What is not admitted in any women's magazines is that these same magazines published forty-five articles promoting breast implants between 1980 and 1989.

The sole article criticizing the media's role in promoting medical solutions to women's appearance concerns appeared in a 1994 *Glamour*. Its focus, however, is on television and newspaper reports of a Mayo Clinic study of 749 women with implants, published in the *New England Journal of Medicine* that year. The author notes that the Mayo researchers appropriately acknowledge that they were only looking for systemic diseases—diseases spread through the lymph system or bloodstream—and would need a much larger sample to detect increased risk of rarer connective-tissue diseases. Moreover, the women were followed for only an average of 7.8 years, too short a time to determine chronic effects. The author chastises newspaper and television reporters for failing to mention these important limitations to the research findings. Instead, from the *New York Times* to the *Dallas Morning News*, reporters proclaimed that the study found no implant-disease links. Since 1995, however, several large-scale studies have reported no significant statistical evidence of autoimmune diseases (Kaiser 1998).

The marketing of cosmetic surgery in women's magazines continues to increase. A new magazine designed specifically for women interested in cosmetic surgery, *Form and Figure: The Future of Beauty*, debuted in 1998. The ASPRS targeted women's magazines in its 1997 and 1998 national campaigns to advertise cosmetic procedures. Following the successful strategy of pharmaceutical companies, manufacturers of cosmetic surgery devices began advertising directly to consumers in mid-1999. The first ads were for breast implants and were placed in women's magazines and on television and radio. The number of breast implant surgeries are once again increasing rapidly.

8 | Pandora's Box

Commercialism in the Medical Profession

Commercialism is a powerful force in American society. The emphasis on producing profits in competitive markets has led to greater efficiencies of production and marketing strategies designed to increase demand. These efficiencies have lowered the costs of many goods and services and elevated the material well-being of the average person. American bodies are fed, cleaned, clothed, decorated, medicated, housed, transported, entertained, waked, and buried by commercial goods and services. Advertising for these products permeates our culture. Profit-driven commercial hype is so pervasive that adults regard it as another fact of life to teach children in our affluent consumer culture.

There has always been money to be made in medicine. Yet, we do not include physicians in our warnings about marketing hype because we usually do not think of their work with patients as a commercial trade. The American Medical Association (AMA) drove commercialism out of the physician-patient relationship in its campaign to establish the professional authority and autonomy of physicians at the beginning of the twentieth century. Other than the pharmaceutical and insurance industries, there was little commercialism in medicine for about two-thirds of the twentieth century. Solo practitioners tended their patients in their own offices and at nonprofit community hospitals. They were paid either out of the patients' own pockets or by the patients' health insurance companies; approximately half of these patients were covered by the nonprofit Blue Cross–Blue Shield. But, blatant commercialism returned to medicine. It has spread beyond the pharmaceutical and medical equipment industries to nursing homes, hospitals, labs, and clinics and now dominates the insurance industry and the corporate delivery of health services. A competitive, commercial sector has emerged within clinical medicine as well, and cosmetic surgery is at its cutting edge. After briefly highlighting the main findings of the previous chapters, I will discuss the implications of commercialism in medicine for patients and the medical profession.

A Sociological Perspective

This book started with the premise that cosmetic surgery, as a modern body custom, has social meaning worth exploring because social bodies provide clues to the dynamics of the larger culture and social structures. What meaning we discover depends on which path we explore. Some have examined the influence of popular culture on the history of cosmetic surgery (Gilman 1999; Haiken 1997). Others have examined what patients and practitioners say about cosmetic surgery (Davis 1995; Dull and West 1991). In contrast, I have explored several paths that led to a macro-level understanding of cosmetic surgery as a modern body custom rather than an individual's body choice. Consequently, I have nothing additional to offer to the debate about whether an individual's decision to have cosmetic surgery is a form of self-empowerment and self-healing, an unconscious compliance with gendered cultural pressures, or a consciously risky choice driven by vanity or low self-esteem.

I offer a sociological explanation of cosmetic surgery, not a psychological one. It begins with the increasingly narrow definition of a desirable appearance, which is driven by media innovations that have saturated the culture with body images. It includes the social, psychological, and economic advantages and disadvantages that are connected with the master status of appearance, consequences that have been exacerbated by structural changes in the economy, employment, and families. The malleable nature of appearance has made cosmetic surgery a strategy for upward social mobility for some patients.

Patient demand is not sufficient to create a medical practice. Physicians must participate. Therefore, my explanation of cosmetic surgery as a body custom necessarily has to include the structural changes affecting the supply of practitioners willing to do cosmetic operations.

These include changes within medicine and at the intersection between medicine and other major social institutions, including the economy and the government. Cosmetic surgery was made possible by technological changes in medicine developed to restore function and form to the disfigured. It became a more common body custom when the supply of physicians exceeded demand for traditional reconstructive work, training in cosmetic techniques became more readily available, and surgery began to move out of hospitals. It became a highly competitive area of medicine when its potential financial rewards and lack of third-party oversight attracted physicians from other areas of medicine where corporatization and privatization threaten their economic well-being and sense of professional autonomy. It became a commercial product when a series of court decisions eroded the traditional distinction between the "learned professions" and other trades under antitrust law and the Federal Trade Commission (FTC) forced state licensure boards and professional associations to deregulate their marketing restrictions in a policy aimed at reducing the spiraling costs of health care.

Physicians originally fought the deregulation of medical marketing. Some have since been seduced by the power of commercialism, unleashed by deregulation. Nowhere are ethical concerns about supplier-induced demand and conflict of interest more legitimate than in commercially offered physician services such as cosmetic surgery. Commercialism, like Pandora's box, is full of problems for the medical profession's service ethic, occupational authority, and autonomy.

Service Ethic Challenged

Unlike a commercial trade, medicine has a service ethic that prohibits the exploitation of patients for profit. This service ethic, along with specialized knowledge, forms the foundation on which organized medicine's legitimacy as a profession rests. It also is the foundation of the trust that characterizes a good patient-physician relationship and counterbalances the asymmetry of knowledge between the two. Service to the needs of others, rather than maximization of personal gain, is an essential element of a true profession.

In the case of cosmetic surgery, the distinction between medicine and other commercial trades is not as clear as it once was. Like other commercial trades, many, if not most, physicians who offer cosmetic surgery now use both advertising and public relations to boost demand for their work. Like the marketing of other commercial goods and services, the pitch for cosmetic surgery appeals to the dominant cultural values of youth, beauty, sexuality, status, happiness, and control. It exploits people's anxieties and fantasies. It ignores the social origins of demand and personalizes the problem of perceived appearance imperfections. It emphasizes positive outcomes and downplays the pain and risks of medical intervention. Claims of expertise, ease, safety, and desirable outcomes are occasionally exaggerated to the point of misrepresentation to increase sales. Sometimes prospective patients are persuaded to expand their perception of their appearance problems. Sometimes they are pressured to commit to surgery by offers of discounts for an immediate decision or for multiple procedures. Such sales-building practices are expected in other commercial businesses from retail and restaurants to real estate. In medicine, however, they raise ethical questions about the exploitation of vulnerable patients by those who have a fiduciary responsibility to act in patients' best interests. These questions, in turn, make the profession's service ethic vulnerable to public challenge.

A 1998 investigative series of newspaper articles on cosmetic surgery in Florida by the *Sun-Sentinel* (Schulte and Bergal 1998) provides an example of a public challenge to physicians' service ethic. The series was a finalist for a Pulitzer prize. Cosmetic surgery is a booming business in Florida. More than one of every ten procedures in the country by board-certified plastic surgeons takes place in Florida (American Society of Plastic and Reconstructive Surgeons 1999d). Only California has substantially more. New York has about the same number. Facial plastic surgeons and other practicing cosmetic surgeons also are in abundance in these three states. Florida, however, has a much smaller population than the other two states, making it the most active cosmetic surgery market in the country.

Most patients in Florida are happy with their cosmetic outcomes, but not all. *Sun-Sentinel* reporters spent six months examining the state's malpractice insurance claims, lawsuits, newspaper accounts, medical examiner autopsy reports, Board of Medicine disciplinary reports, police reports, and other public documents. They uncovered thirty-four deaths (subsequently revised to thirty-nine) related to cosmetic surgery between 1986 and the first quarter of 1999. Eighteen of the deaths occurred in the most recent twenty-six months. The reporters and the experts they interviewed readily admitted there may have been more.

The causes of death ranged from anesthesia overdoses and blood clots in the lungs to cardiac arrhythmia and fecal peritonitis caused by perforation of the abdominal wall. A three-year-old died undergoing office-based laser treatments for "port wine stains" by a former emergency room physician who had no oxygen available. A sixty-six-year-old woman with a history of high blood pressure died after thirteen pounds of fat and skin were removed during six hours of liposuction in an office facility. An overweight sixty-two-year-old woman with significant hardening of the arteries and high blood pressure stopped breathing after nine hours of facial surgery in an office facility. A fifty-one-year-old man died while spending the night at a physician's office after almost ten hours of surgery during which he had a facelift, liposuction around his waist, and fat injected into his penis.

The *Sun-Sentinel* reporters looked for trends in the 810 malpractice insurance claims filed between 1986 and 1998. The insurance companies judged about 40 percent to involve serious permanent damage after reviewing each patient's medical record. They had already paid $38.2 million in compensation. The nature of the claims varied widely. A young man was compensated for disfigurement and disability after his pectoral implants became painfully infected. Others have been compensated for severe burns from laser treatments to remove wrinkles and for disfigurement from abdominoplasty, breast implants, and other procedures. Claims can take years to resolve. The case of a female personal trainer left comatose after liposuction to remove minor amounts of fat remains open at the time of this writing as all medical personnel involved dispute responsibility. She went into cardiac arrest during the procedure and was revived by paramedics and an anesthesiologist who were called to the office by staff. After they left, her physician resumed the operation. She never regained consciousness and has been diagnosed with severe brain damage. Another liposuction case involved a woman who awoke in pain during an overnight office stay to find no one present. She crawled outside where she collapsed. She spent five days in intensive care.

These injuries and deaths illustrate three broad problems with cosmetic surgery. All stem from its commercial, free-market delivery system. First, deregulation of marketing has made cosmetic surgery a potentially lucrative business, dependent on marketing. One in four plastic surgeons nationwide had a net income of $300,000 or more in 1997. Achieving such high profits depends on attracting a high volume of patients; this, in turn, requires making a substantial investment in promotion. The *Sun-Sentinel* reporters quoted a physician who said,

"Trying to turn out case after case to meet your advertising budget is a very bad thing for this business. It can be harmful." The more competitive the market is, the more aggressive and questionable some marketing campaigns are. Another physician warned, "Let the buyer beware. . . . The seductive, unbelievably unrealistic balloon of fantasy is floated out there, promulgated by the media." The reporters concluded that many of the two hundred Florida ads they looked at stretched the rules against false and misleading advertising. One egregious example, a full-page ad in their own newspaper, offered "guaranteed painless procedures" by a physician who had at least one cosmetic patient die in his care. The physician claimed his ad was not misleading because patients experience no pain during anesthetized procedures, only afterwards.

Like some other states, Florida has had a surge of cosmetic surgery facilities opened by nonphysicians looking for high profits. These investors have no personal stake in maintaining the profession's ethical standards. They pay salaried or, more often, freelancing physicians to operate on patients they recruit with aggressive advertising campaigns and aggressive sales staffs, often paid on commission. One owner, a convicted burglar, claimed he paid his female staff a 20 to 25 percent commission. Their sales pitch for breast implants included displaying their own to prospective patients, who, he acknowledged to the *Sun-Sentinel* reporters, included more "strippers" than "society types." Offers of discounts for multiple procedures or immediate commitment are common both at these investor-owned facilities and at physician-owned facilities. As a result, more patients spend more time under anesthesia, raising the risks correspondingly. When complications occur, many complain they were pressured into surgery and not informed about risks.

A second source of problems is the minimal state regulation of surgery in private office facilities. State health authorities and legislators are generally unaware of the extent of the problem. Most states lack regulations for the most basic kinds of monitoring of office surgery. Like every other state except New Jersey, Florida does not require physicians operating outside of hospitals and surgicenters to report deaths and serious complications. As a result, the risks are hidden from health authorities and potential patients. Like every other state except California, Florida does not require offices where surgery takes place to be accredited or even inspected. As a result, some facilities lack proper aseptic conditions or are ill-equipped to deal with serious complications. Office staffs sometimes lack credentials to assist in surgery or to care for patients during recovery. There are no record-keeping requirements. Like every other state except New Jersey, Florida does not impose specific restrictions on patient screening, the types of procedures that can be done, or the duration of office surgery. As a result, in this competitive environment physicians are free to push the limits of good medical judgement. Some accept patients whose medical history, age, or behaviors, such as smoking, put them at higher risk. Some keep patients under anesthesia in ill-equipped and inadequately staffed offices for as long as heart or kidney transplant patients in hospitals where regulations are strict. Lengthy operations greatly increase the risks of complications for even the lowest-risk patients.

A third source of problems is lax oversight of individual physicians' practices by their own licensure boards. Like every other state, Florida has few barriers to an office-based surgical practice. As a result, practitioners with little or no supervised experience in cosmetic surgery, no formal training in plastic techniques, and even no formal training in surgery can take up cosmetic surgery. One testified in court that he taught himself liposuction by experimenting on a pig and subsequently taught others. Like many other states, Florida's understaffed Board of Medicine contends with a large backlog of potential disciplinary cases that take an average of nineteen to forty months to resolve. As a result, in most cases physicians continue to practice for years while the question of their medical judgement or competence is undecided. Like most other states, Florida's Board of Medicine rarely revokes a physician's license to practice. Even in cases where the board finds clear evidence of a substandard medical practice linked to deaths and serious injuries, most disciplinary outcomes are limited to temporary suspensions and fines, small by comparison with the typical cost of one or two cosmetic surgeries.

State licensure boards only investigate cases where a complaint is filed. There is little other monitoring of medical outcomes. Like other states, medical examiners in some Florida districts do not routinely investigate surgical deaths, in or out of hospitals, because they lack sufficient resources. When they do review cases, the medical examiners usually rule that deaths during and after surgery from anesthesia, lacerated arteries, and the like are due to "natural causes" because these injuries are known risks of surgery. The only other recourse when care is substandard or negligent is a malpractice suit. Like other states,

Florida does not require physicians to carry malpractice insurance. As a result, patients can find themselves without meaningful recourse when a physician decides not to carry insurance and declares bankruptcy.

Board-certified plastic surgeons interviewed by *Sun-Sentinel reporters* attribute Florida's cosmetic surgery problems to unqualified competitors. One claimed that "Florida has become the dust bin for any incompetent in the country." The reporters' investigation did find malpractice claims against a few physicians who took up cosmetic surgery after experiencing malpractice actions in other specialties. Nevertheless, they report that more than 80 percent of Florida's physicians with multiple medical malpractice claims for deaths and serious injuries are board-certified in plastic surgery. Plastic surgeons have the fourth-highest rate of malpractice claims in the state.

Officials at the Department of Health and members of the Board of Medicine reacted strongly to the reporters' findings. A physician-administrator at the Department of Health told reporters, "This really is something that is getting way out of control. This is a money-driven area (of medicine), and it is getting worse and worse. . . . You're no more than a merchant. You're a business. You might as well have double Green Stamp days. . . . I never in my wildest dreams would have thought people would be staying in the doctor's office for 24 hours." He urged legislators to adopt some regulations to protect patients.

Most physicians value their professional privileges and practice responsibly and ethically to uphold the public's trust and maintain their professional authority and autonomy. Their conscientious efforts, however, can be eclipsed when the reckless practices of a few colleagues are brought to the public's attention. As we have seen in recent years with politicians and lawyers, the public tends to impute the questionable behavior of a few individuals to the group. There is also the tendency for the actions of the minority who are pushing the borders of responsible and ethical practice to change the norms of acceptable practice. This is clearly evident in the increasing duration of office surgeries. As Mark Gorney, a former president of the American Society of Plastic and Reconstructive Surgeons (ASPRS) who fought hard to overturn the FTC's decision to deregulate all but deceptive and false advertising, told the *Sun-Sentinel* reporters, "This will end badly. There's just too much cash on the barrel. When we started out, we were doctors first. One tends to forget that you took an oath to first do no harm."

Authority Challenged

Patients have long trusted the ancient Hippocratic oath to protect them. A former patient interviewed by the *Sun-Sentinel* reporters illustrates how thoroughly dependent most patients are on physicians' ethics. The woman was left with a grossly deformed abdomen after surgery by a general surgeon who advertised "the most advanced cosmetic surgery procedures and techniques." She said, "I never asked him if he had the qualifications. I was from the old school. You believe your doctor. Boy, did I get a rude awakening." When the media give a public voice to patients who question their personal physicians' competence and ethics, the profession's authority is challenged.

This was not the first time that American physicians engaged in cosmetic surgery had their authority challenged. Beauty surgeons in the early twentieth century found themselves under attack from both journalists and regular physicians who were determined to eliminate commercialism from medicine. Chapter 3 discusses the vitriolic campaign against commercialism and for public legitimation of professional authority, a campaign that eventually drove cosmetic surgery into the medical closet.

Another national attack on the authority of physicians engaged in cosmetic surgery occurred around the time of the 1989 congressional hearings, "Unqualified Doctors Performing Cosmetic Surgery: Policies and Enforcement: Activities of the Federal Trade Commission" (U.S. House 1989a,b,c), discussed in chapter 5. Board-certified plastic surgeons tried to use these hearings to generate legislation to reverse the FTC's deregulation of medical marketing that had swelled the competition for cosmetic surgery patients. They encountered strong opposition from their fellow-physician rivals who claimed that board-certified plastic surgeons were less concerned with patient protection than with turf protection. Board-certified plastic surgeons failed to present statistical evidence of outcomes superior to their rivals and lacked the support of the AMA to counter the appeal of their rivals' antitrust arguments.

Less than a year later plastic surgeons and others engaged in cosmetic surgery were back in Washington. This time they were called to answer questions during the hearing, "Is the FDA Protecting Patients from the Dangers of Silicone Breast Implants?" (U.S. House 1990). The breast implant controversy that followed (discussed in chapters 4 and 7) often portrayed them and their rivals as "money-grubbing cosmetic surgeons" rather than altruistic healers whose authority could be trusted. The ASPRS spent a considerable amount of money on public relations to repair the damage to plastic surgeons' reputations.

At the time of this writing the strongest public challenge to the authority of plastic surgeons and others engaged in cosmetic surgery is in Florida. New Jersey recently adopted a few regulatory measures to curb some office-based surgery risks. A few other states, including California and New York, are beginning to discuss the problems of unregulated office-based cosmetic surgery. California declared a moratorium on large-volume liposuctions after a highly publicized recent death. Depending on the outcome of the ongoing attempts to restrict the practice of office-based cosmetic practitioners in Florida, the challenge to the authority and ultimately the autonomy of office-based cosmetic practitioners could expand into a national movement.

Autonomy Challenged

At least some cosmetic practitioners express resentment at the social, economic, and political changes which, they claim, force them to expand their work beyond those patients whose appearance concerns they judge to be legitimate. After meeting a woman in her late sixties whose lifted face looked much younger than the rest of her body, the editor of *Plastic and Reconstructive Surgery* wondered if "[o]ur technical prowess may outstrip our aesthetic judgement" (Goldwyn 1990b, 949). He expressed similar reservations about colleagues who lift the faces of women in their thirties and suggested that these operations may be a surgical version of the "Emperor's New Clothes." He added, "Knowing when to stop in surgery is a hard lesson to learn. Knowing when to begin may be even harder." Others have also worried that practitioners have been "forced to compromise good surgical judgement for the sake of lucre" (Kisner 1993, 1364).

The free exercise of medical judgement is at the heart of professional medicine. This includes physicians' right to refuse to provide treatments that they believe are ineffective or have potential benefits too limited to justify the risks, even when informed patients want the treatments and can pay for them. Fear of losing this professional autonomy is the primary reason that organized medicine resisted salaried employment, resisted a national health insurance program, resisted Medicare and Medicaid, resisted managed care, resisted peer and administrative review, and now resists the intrusion of finance companies and other nonmedical investors in medicine and attempts by governments and licensure boards to regulate their practices.

Physicians' autonomy rests on their expertise and their fiduciary relationship with patients, a relationship that is strained by the emphasis on profit that is inherent in commercialism. Physicians who invest money to attract patients in any of the ways previously discussed, or who work as independent contractors for others, undoubtedly feel pressure to accept the patients who come to them and to piggyback cosmetic procedures. Nevertheless, all claim to turn away prospective patients whom they judge to be inappropriate candidates for surgery. They also claim to decline to perform procedures or multiple procedures that they judge to be inappropriate. Where each physician draws the line between appropriate and inappropriate varies, but only the existence of this thin line of expert judgement now separates commercial medicine from other businesses where the principle of caveat emptor, rather than professional trust, rules. In highly competitive markets, such as in Florida, this line has become a slippery slope.

Whether physicians' expert judgement can be trusted when it comes to cosmetic surgery in the privacy of their offices has been the subject of contentious debate in Florida since the *Sun-Sentinel* published its investigative series. Within a few weeks, a state legislator introduced two bills. The first had provisions to strengthen the Board of Medicine's regulatory authority and require state inspection of office surgical facilities. It also would have required confidential reports of serious injuries and deaths related to office-based surgery to alert health authorities to problem physicians and problem practices. The second bill would have required ads to include information about the risks of cosmetic surgery. At the same time, the Board of Medicine unanimously voted in favor of imposing restrictions on office-based surgery, restrictions that would severely curtail physicians' judgmental autonomy. The proposed regulations included

- A mandatory report of deaths and serious injuries within 15 days;
- A four-hour limit on surgery;
- A physician-anesthesiologist must administer or supervise anesthesia;
- A four-pound limit on fat removal;
- A ban on overnight stays;
- Accreditation of surgical facilities by a nationally recognized organization or inspection by the state.

The Board of Medicine's proposed regulations could not go into effect before a public hearing for comment from all interested parties. The reaction of interested physicians was swift and pugnacious.

As board members anticipated, and the *Sun-Sentinel* reported, those involved with cosmetic surgery did "everything possible to torpedo what we've achieved so far." They waged an aggressive offense to preserve their autonomy. Even the small sixty-member Florida Academy of Cosmetic Surgery hired a powerful lobbyist. Nurse-anesthetists joined the fight. Hundreds of individual physicians wrote to protest the "knee-jerk response to the media." They argued that the limits on the duration of surgery and fat removal were based on anecdotal reports rather than scientific data. They argued that nurse-anesthetists, who administer most office-based anesthesia for about half the fee of anesthesiologists, were fully competent to work under an operating physician's supervision. They argued that "all the laws in the world won't change bad judgement" and that the board should leave medical decision-making to those doing the specialty work. Instead of passing regulations that would undermine the autonomy of physicians, they suggested that the board concentrate on weeding out incompetent and reckless physicians.

Board-certified plastic surgeons, many of whom had built elaborate surgical facilities with recovery suites, strenuously objected to the ban on overnight stays. They claimed their facilities exposed patients to fewer risks of infection than hospitals and provided better care than homes or hotel rooms. Additionally, they argued that the ban would increase the risk of complications by forcing them to push patients out their offices prematurely. The plastic surgeons lobbied to require physicians to have hospital privileges for the cosmetic procedures they do in offices, a stipulation vehemently opposed by their rivals, who claimed that plastic surgeons on hospital staffs block their requests for privileges.

The legislature passed a modified version of the first bill, a version that dropped the provisions to strengthen the regulatory authority of the Board of Medicine and to require state inspections. Defending the compromise, the bill's sponsor told *Sun-Sentinel* reporters, "If you knew how much lobbying there was in the last two weeks and the amount of money that went into it, you'd be shocked that we got this passed."

The Board of Medicine's public hearing on its proposed regulations turned into an acrimonious six-hour session. More than 150 physicians attended. Only one former patient was allowed to testify. Under heavy attack, the now divided board, with three new appointees, re-treated. The restriction on surgery time was extended to six hours. The restriction on fat removal was increased to five pounds. The require-ment that an anesthesiologist supervise or directly administer anes-thesia was deleted. The plastic surgeons temporarily won their battle to mandate that physicians who operate with general anesthesia have hospital privileges to perform the same operations they do in offices. In response to claims that the ban on overnight stays in offices would increase patient risks, the board added a requirement that physicians arrange adequate postoperative care for their patients. The compromises did not satisfy anyone.

Only twelve hours after the hearing, the board revisited the regu-lations and retreated further. The revised regulations for office-based surgery eliminated the hospital privileges requirement, loosened other requirements, and added a few substitutes:

- A mandatory report of deaths and serious injuries within 15 days;
- An eight-hour limit on surgery;
- A nine-pound limit on fat removal;
- A restriction on overnight stays to 23 hours;
- Accreditation of surgical facilities by a nationally recognized or-ganization or inspection by the state;
- A registered nurse and an assistant must be present in recovery rooms;
- Patients must be fully informed about potential risks;
- Physicians must have some surgical training in the procedures they perform.

A consumer member of the board told reporters, "This really distresses me. Doctors have demonstrated they don't have common sense. They make economic decisions. It's basically the wild west out there."

The issue is far from over at this time. Three hospital groups filed a legal challenge to the new regulations. They claimed the rules will compromise patient safety and authorize minimally regulated hospi-tals in physicians' offices. One administrator noted that physicians could offer open-heart surgery in their offices under these rules. Nev-ertheless, these rules would be the strictest in the country. The board anticipates more legal challenges from physician groups opposed to any infringement on their professional autonomy. The Florida Acad-emy of Cosmetic Surgery has already requested another public hear-ing to clarify the rules. They are probably concerned that board-certified

plastic surgeons can use the surgical training requirement to drive them
out of the cosmetic surgery business. Whether Florida's Board of Medicine will succeed in asserting any control over office surgery remains
to be seen.

A Caveat about Victims and Villains

Perhaps because individual responsibility is a
dominant ideology in American culture, we tend to personalize problems. Heart disease and strokes are attributed to poor diet, inadequate
exercise, and smoking. AIDS is blamed on engaging in risky, promis-
cuous sex and intravenous drug use. Teenage pregnancy is linked to
a lack of moral values and self-control. These explanations blame individuals for their health needs and mask the role of social institutions and the culture in shaping dietary choices, exercise habits,
smoking, and sexual behavior. Undoubtedly, some readers of the
Sun-Sentinel similarly interpreted the cosmetic surgery articles as a
parable about foolish patients driven to reckless behavior because of
vanity or low self-esteem and unethical physicians driven to reckless
behavior because of greed or arrogance. This moral interpretation casts
the patients as victims and the physicians as villains and overlooks
the secular social arrangements that created this body custom.

If the story of cosmetic surgery has to have a victim, I would argue that both patients and physicians qualify for the role. Prospective
patients are well aware that there are strong stereotypes connected with
appearance and that these stereotypes have significant social and economic effects. They are as potentially vulnerable as any consumers to
the power of marketing. Marketing sells products and services by as-
sociating them, literally or symbolically, with dominant cultural ideologies, values, and beliefs. To market cosmetic surgery, beauty, sexual
allure, control, power, affluence, and youth are presented as achieved
rather than ascribed characteristics. Surgical self-improvement is sold
as the ticket to upward social mobility and high self-esteem. The possibilities of poor aesthetic outcomes, short-term effects, health risks,
and costs are downplayed. Medical consumers have little post-purchase
recourse. There are no returns and no money-back guarantees if outcomes fail to live up to patients' expectations. Most are happy with
their outcomes. Those who are not either undergo additional surgery
or learn to live with the repercussions of their choices. In the worst
cases, they or their surviving family members file complaints with
medical boards and sue their practitioners.

Physicians also have been victimized by cosmetic surgery. They did not ask the courts or the FTC to deregulate restrictions on marketing professional services. They vehemently opposed it, claiming that the commercialization of medicine would have dire consequences for some patients' health. The Supreme Court decisions that paved the way for commercialization reveal strong reservations among some justices about injecting commercialism into a profession with a fiduciary responsibility to a group as vulnerable as patients. Despite these legitimate reservations and considerable political clout, the AMA failed to convince Congress to exempt physicians from the jurisdiction of the FTC. The AMA was unable to overcome the deregulatory dogma of the Reagan era.

The resulting added competition for cosmetic patients has intensified the level of commercialization and its related problems. Most cosmetic patients fare well, but a few, as we have seen in the case of Florida, have the kinds of disastrous outcomes that opponents of marketing deregulation predicted. Most physicians practice responsibly, but a few, as we have seen in the case of Florida, have been corrupted by commercialism's emphasis on maximizing profits, even at the expense of patient safety. Their behavior undermines the profession's status and threatens its occupational privileges.

If both patients and physicians are victims, who are the villains? In the story of cosmetic surgery, there are two main villains, but they are not people. One is our ideas about appearance. Our preference for people with facial and body symmetry and average or exaggerated sex-linked features may have some biological underpinnings, as discussed in chapter 2, but culture fleshes out our gender-specific ideal body standards. We saw, in chapter 1, that these standards are remodeled in response to social change. This connection between body standards and social institutions, ideologies, values, and beliefs gives appearance cultural meaning and social consequences. The cultural meanings of various appearances lead to stereotypic expectations and differential treatment in everyday life. The villainy of our ideas about appearance is that they diminish less attractive people's opportunities to maximize their own potential and, consequently, their contributions to society. It is a lose-lose outcome. Therefore, the consequences of appearance discrimination are not merely personal problems, they are political problems, just like the consequences of discrimination based on other master statuses such as gender, race, ethnicity, age, and religion. The energy we spend on surveillance of our body imperfections could be better spent working for social change to reduce the origin and social impact of prejudices about appearance.

The other villain in the cosmetic surgery story is the commercialization of medicine. To understand what makes commercialism in medicine problematic, we need to reflect on the meaning of the concept. Commercialism, according to *Webster's Ninth New Collegiate Dictionary,* is an "excessive emphasis on profit," and "exploit for profit." The term commercial is synonymous with "average or inferior quality" and refers to something that is "designed for a large market," and "supported by advertisers." Advertising also can be used to create a perception of "need" for newly created services and products, a need that can be exploited for profit. A few health examples include treatments for halitosis, dandruff, mood elevation, lethargy, and height. While not all commercial products are highly profitable, mass produced, of inferior quality, and of questionable value, these dictionary definitions point to the slippery slope of compromised ethics and quality often found in for-profit commerce.

Commercialism is not a new development. The principle of caveat emptor has been used in business since at least 1523 to remind buyers that they assume some risk of poor quality when they make unwarranted purchases. Unwarranted purchases are the norm in medicine; the outcomes of medical treatment are not as predictable as most other goods and services. There are always risks of complications and poor outcomes, even in the simplest interventions by adequately trained, responsible practitioners. In the hands of less cautious practitioners who have been lured down the slippery slope of compromised quality by the prospect of higher profits, complications and poor outcomes multiply.

The Future of Commercialism in Medicine

Cosmetic surgery may be on the cutting edge of commercial medicine in America, but it is not alone. Elective treatments for vision, snoring, infertility, impotency, and weight control are a few other areas of medicine aggressively marketed by physicians. Many other types of practitioners from acupuncturists and chiropractors to dentists and homeopaths also advertise their services.

Some areas of health care have always been commercial. Pharmaceutical and medical equipment corporations have always relied heavily on advertising. These for-profit enterprises have a long history of using creative marketing strategies to sell their over-the-counter products. Following the creation of a restricted class of drugs and other products, they developed additional strategies aimed at physicians. Their considerable marketing budgets subsidize many medical journals and professional conferences. Their "detail" men and women wine and dine individual physicians willing to listen to their sales pitches. They host physicians and their spouses at company-sponsored conferences in places like Hawaii. They pay physicians to participate in research studies.

These monetary ties raise concern that this medical-industrial complex insidiously manipulates physicians' treatment decisions in ways that enhance corporate profits and inflate the country's health care costs. The commercial nature of drug companies raises another concern that their profit-driven focus on mass markets yields too many similar drugs for common health problems and too few breakthrough drugs for rare diseases. Legislation to induce "orphan drug" research has not solved this problem. Concern also has been raised by court cases that reveal some companies have concealed information about adverse reactions from the Food and Drug Administration (FDA) in their zeal to seize or maintain a large share of the market for their products. These concerns have taken a new urgency with the FDA's recent relaxation of restrictions on marketing prescription drugs directly to the public and the increasing availability of those drugs on the Internet. Ads for drugs to treat allergies, arthritis, depression, anxiety, flu, impotence, birth control, menopause, heart disease, and other common problems have exploded into a $1 billion market (*Advertising Age* 1998). This development raises the prospect that supplier-induced demand will increase health care costs without additional therapeutic effects and will inevitably result in more adverse outcomes.

The incursion of commercialism in other areas of health care has also been problematic. After Medicare and Medicaid legislation in the mid-1960s provided funding for elderly and indigent health care, investors built nursing home chains to capture profits from the economies of larger scale and more economically efficient management of resources. The latter has expanded to include screening out sicker patients who need more services, favoring higher-paying private patients over lower-paying Medicaid patients, and staffing with mostly unskilled, low-paid workers. The questionable quality of care for the frail, sick residents in some of these facilities has been a reoccurring topic for investigative reporters around the country and has led to tighter government regulation of the industry. (Changes in Medicare reimbursement policies have since pushed the most recklessly managed nursing home corporations into Chapter 11 bankruptcy. At the beginning of 2000, these companies owned about 10 percent of the country's nursing homes.)

Persistent concerns that some commercial nursing homes abuse their fiduciary relationship with vulnerable patients did not stop the financial success of this industry in the 1970s from propelling the commercialization and corporate integration of hospitals. The infusion of large amounts of investors' money resulted in the rapid demise of many small, independent, nonprofit, community hospitals. The majority of remaining hospitals are still nonprofit, although many are corporately linked to for-profit facilities and services. These nonprofit ones survived the new competition only by forming multi-hospital corporate structures like the for-profit ones and by adopting similar business practices. These practices include dumping uninsured patients on public hospitals, closing unprofitable services, marketing profitable services like maternity care, and running up the bills of patients with "fee-for-service" insurance.

As a result, medical care costs continued to climb, despite the anticipated economic efficiencies of corporatization and privatization in the hospital industry. The government responded with new regulations. In the early 1980s it restructured payment for in-patient care under Medicare and Medicaid to replace the inflationary incentive of the previous fee-for-service system with a capitated fee-for-diagnosis system. Many private insurance companies adopted similar types of reimbursement. Controlling costs in this increasingly commercial industry has proven difficult. Hospitals shifted a large portion of surgery and other services to outpatient facilities and released admitted patients "sicker and quicker." Some of these patients go to step-down and rehabilitation facilities run by the same corporation, which can bill separately for the services at a different facility. These hospital corporations also unbundled other profitable services, such as diagnostic laboratories, to maximize billing.

The insurance industry has similarly undergone considerable commercialization since the late 1970s. Prior to that, the nonprofit Blue Cross–Blue Shield indemnity programs dominated the market for forty years, despite competing with more than one thousand commercial firms. Lack of cost containment ultimately toppled the reign of the "Blues." Widespread corporate frustration with the soaring cost of employee health benefits and increased government incentives eventually enticed private investors to set up managed care programs that combined insurance coverage with the delivery of health services in the 1980s. These programs usually offer more health care coverage for less cost by using their buying power to negotiate lower fees, eliminating unnecessary care, substituting more cost-effective care, financially rewarding physicians who use fewer resources on patients, and otherwise rationing services, particularly those of hospitals and specialists. Most managed care companies were profitable in the 1980s and 1990s partly because there was considerable excess usage under fee-for-service reimbursement. They will have a difficult time maintaining the same level of profits in the future because both physicians and patients increasingly complain that these commercial managed-care corporations provide inferior-quality care.

The search for profit in a competitive consumer product market can lead to higher-quality, more reliable, lower-cost goods such as televisions, automobiles, computers, and refrigerators. In contrast, the search for profit in a fiduciary service such as medicine can lead to ethically compromising behavior that erodes trust. This is why the AMA fought to eradicate commercialism from medicine at the beginning of the twentieth century and sought an exemption from FTC oversight in the early 1980s. Nevertheless, the AMA's own actions in 1997 demonstrate that no person and no organization is invulnerable to the powerful temptation of commercialism.

Faced with declining revenues from dues, the AMA agreed to place its professional seal on Sunbeam's heating pads, humidifiers, and other "Health at Home" products in exchange for anticipated millions of dollars in royalties on sales. By agreeing to "co-brand" or "rent" the well-known icon of its reputation to raise money, the AMA embraced a practice that has become common among national health charities such as the American Cancer Association and the American Heart Association. For the most part, these arrangements have aroused little public complaint.

The AMA's arrangement, in contrast, provoked impassioned protest from individual physicians and their specialty associations and a lambasting by consumer advocates, academic ethicists, and editorialists across the country, at least one of whom called it the prostitution of the profession's public trust. The uproar forced the dismissals and resignations of the executives directly responsible for the agreement. It also forced the association to renege on the contract, prompting Sunbeam to sue. To avoid more legal costs and negative publicity (a Louis

Harris and Associates survey found that only 13 percent of the public was aware of the scandal), the AMA settled the suit, paying almost $10 million (Klein 1998). It was a costly mistake for the association, but it could have been worse. The FDA has since castigated Sunbeam's quality assurance procedures for some of the same products that the AMA was going to endorse. Following the fiasco, the AMA adopted a strategic plan aimed at restoring its credibility both as the "acknowledged leader in setting standards for medical ethics, practice and education" and as the "most authoritative voice and influential advocate for physicians and their patients" (*American Medical News* 1999).

We no longer have just the nose of commercialism in the medical tent, we have the whole camel. Restraining its temptations will be a difficult task to accomplish internally, given the increasing fragmentation and competition within medicine and the weakened voice and power of the AMA. As long as the government refuses to distinguish between the medical profession and other commercial trades under antitrust law, public oversight and regulations, like those under debate in Florida, will be needed to protect patients. By reining in the most imprudent medical practices, such regulatory oversight also will help protect the profession's reputation.

Bibliography

Abbot, Andrew. 1988. *The System of Professions.* Chicago: University of Chicago Press.

Adamson, Peter. 1998. *The Future of the American Board of Facial Plastic and Reconstructive Surgery.* www.abfprs.org/Announcements.

Advertising Age. 1998. "Prescription for Profit: Direct to Consumer Advertising." 69:S1–S30.

Alloy, Thomas. 1993. "The Developmental Stability of Facial Attractiveness: New Longitudinal Data and a Review." *Merrill Palmer Quarterly* 39:265–278.

American Academy of Cosmetic Surgery. 2000. *Procedures.* www.cosmetic surgery.org.

American Academy of Facial Plastic and Reconstructive Surgery. 1988. *The Face Book: The Pros and Cons of Facial Plastic Surgery.* Washington, D.C.: Acropolis Books.

———. 1999. *National Statistics on Facial Plastic Surgery.* www.facial-plastic-surgery.org/mediakit/statistics.

American Medical Association. 1971. *Opinions and Reports of the Judicial Council, Including the Principles of Medical Ethics and Rules of the Judicial Council.* Chicago: American Medical Association.

American Medical News. 1977. "FDA Begins 'Trial' of MD Societies." 18(19):21–22.

———. 1997. "Consensus Statement on the Physician Workforce." 40:1, 72, 74.

———. 1999. "The Big Picture: AMA's Strategic Plan for 1999." 42(10): 18.

American Osteopathic Association. 1999. *Media Center.* www.am-osteo-assn.org.

American Society for Aesthetic Plastic Surgery. 1999. www.surgery.org.

———. 2000. www.surgery.org.

American Society for Dermatologic Surgery. 1989. "Testimony." In *Unqualified Doctors Performing Cosmetic Surgery: Policies and Enforcement Activities of the Federal Trade Commission—Part I,* 397–416, House, Committee on Small Business, Subcommittee on Regulation, Business Opportunities, and Energy. 101st Cong., 1st sess.

American Society of Ophthalmic Plastic and Reconstructive Surgery. 1997. *Homepage.* www.asoprs.org/index.html.

American Society of Plastic and Reconstructive Surgeons (ASPRS). 1989a. *Fact Sheet.* Arlington Heights, Ill.: ASPRS.

———. 1989b. *Plastic Surgery Society Calls for Controls on Medical Advertising/Physicians.* Arlington Heights, Ill.: ASPRS.

———. 1996. *A Practical Guide to Marketing Your Plastic Surgery Services to Managed Care.* Arlington Heights, Ill.: ASPRS.

———. 1997. *1997 General Information.* www.plasticssurgery.org/mediactr/97.

———. 1998a. *Cosmetic Surgery Telephone Survey.* www.plasticsurgery.org/mediactr/cossvy.

———. 1998b. *Plastic Surgeons Advise Lipoplasty Patients to Obtain Full Information before Surgery.* Arlington Heights, Ill.: ASPRS.

———. 1999a. *1998 Average Surgeon Fees: Cosmetic and Reconstructive Procedures.* www.plasticsurgery.org/mediactr/98avgsurgfees.

———. 1999b. *1998 Plastic Surgery Procedural Statistics.* www.plasticsurgery.org/mediactr/98statedist.

———. 1999c. *Cosmetic Procedures—Trends 1992, 1996, 1997, 1998.* www.plasticsurgery.org/mediactr/trendsco99.

———. 1999d. *Cosmetic Surgery Jumps 50 percent: Liposuction and Breast Augmentation Top Procedures.* www.plasticsurgery.org/mediactr/99stats.

Anderson, Jack. 1987. "The Plastic Surgery Controversy: Why the Fuss." *Archives of Otolaryngology–Head and Neck Surgery.* 113:709.

Arndt, E., A. Lefebvre, F. Travis, and I. Munro. 1986. "Fact and Fantasy: Psychosocial Consequences of Facial Surgery in 24 Down Syndrome Children." *British Journal of Plastic Surgery* 39:498–504.

Arndt, E., F. Travis, A. Lefebvre, A. Niec, and I. Munro. 1986. "Beauty and the Eye of the Beholder: Social Consequences and Personal Adjustments for Facial Patients." *British Journal of Plastic Surgery* 39:81–84.

Asken, Saul. 1988. *Liposuction Surgery and Autologous Fat Transplantation.* San Mateo, Calif.: Appleton.

Avellone, Joseph, and Francis Moore. 1978. "The Federal Trade Commission Enters a New Arena: Health Services." *New England Journal of Medicine* 299:478–483.

Bailey, Byron. 1987. "Otology—Its Time Has Come!" *Archives of Otolaryngology—Head and Neck Surgery* 113:27–28.

Banner, Lois. 1983. *American Beauty.* Chicago: University of Chicago Press.

Barber, Simon. 1982. "Let's Get Physical: The New Woman's Niche on the Newsstand." *Washington Journalism Review* 4:40–42.

Barry, Ellen. 1998. "Life, Liberty, and the Pursuit of Lipo." *Boston Phoenix,* April 2. www.phx.com/archive/features.

Beaulieu, Anne, and Abby Lippman. 1995. "'Everything You Need to Know' How Women's Magazines Structure Prenatal Diagnosis for Women over 35." *Women and Health* 23:59–74.

Bell, Susan. 1987. "Changing Ideas: The Medicalization of Menopause." *Social Science and Medicine* 24:535–542.

Bettman, Adalbert. 1988. "Plastic and Cosmetic Surgery of the Face." *Aesthetic Plastic Surgery* 12:5–7.

Beuf, Ann Hill. 1990. *Beauty Is the Beast: Appearance-Impaired Children in America.* Philadelphia: University of Pennsylvania Press.

Biddle, Jeff, and Daniel Hamermesh. 1998. "Beauty, Productivity, and Discrimination: Lawyers' Looks and Lucre." *Journal of Labor Economics* 16:172–201.

Blair, Vilary. 1936. "Plastic Surgery of the Head, Face, and Neck: The Psychic Reactions." *Journal of the American Dental Association* 23:236–240.

Bloodgood, Joseph. 1927. "The Possibilities and Dangers of Beauty Operations." *Delineator* 109(10):20ff.

Bogaert, Anthony, and William Fisher. 1995. "Predictors of University Men's Number of Sexual Partners." *Journal of Sex Research* 32:119–130.

Bordo, Susan. 1993. *Unbearable Weight: Feminism, Western Culture, and the Body*. Berkeley: University of California Press.

———. 1997. "Braveheart, Babe, and the Body: Contemporary Images of the Body." In *Twilight Zone: The Hidden Life of Cultural Images from Plato to O. J.*, ed. Susan Bordo. Berkeley: University of California Press.

Brain, Robert. 1979. *The Decorated Body*. London: Hutchinson and Company.

Brody, Garry. 1996a. "Unity Is Plastic Surgery's Strongest Tool." *Plastic Surgery News* 9(4):3.

———. 1996b. "President's Message: Practice Survival Requires Reinvention." *Plastic Surgery News* 9(3):2.

Brown, Jennifer. 1986. "The History of Plastic Surgery: From Ancient India to Modern America." *Bulletin of the American College of Surgeons* 71:21–24.

Brumberg, Joan. 1997. *The Body Project: An Intimate History of American Girls*. New York: Random House.

Bryan, Sharon. 1982. *Pioneering Specialists: History of the American Academy of Ophthalmology and Otolaryngology*. Rochester, Minn.: American Academy of Otolaryngology–Head and Neck Surgery and the American Academy of Ophthalmology.

Burnham, Bruce. 1996. "Notes on the History of the Adoption of Liposuction." *Plastic and Reconstructive Surgery* 97:258–259.

Cameron, K. M., and A. F. Wallace. 1991. "'Dr. Willi' (1882?–1972?), Disciple of Jacques Joseph." *Plastic and Reconstructive Surgery* 88:363–364.

Carter, Lydia, Melanie Hicks, and Steve Slane. 1996. "Women's Reactions to Hypothetical Male Sexual Touch as a Function of Initiator Attractiveness and Level of Coercion." *Sex Roles* 35:737–750.

Casey, Rita, and Jean Ritter. 1996. "How Infant Appearance Informs: Child Care Providers' Responses to Babies Varying in Appearance of Age and Attractiveness." *Journal of Applied Developmental Psychology* 17:495–518.

Cash, Thomas F. 1997. *The Body Image Workbook: An Eight-Step Program for Learning to Like Your Looks*. Oakland, Calif.: New Harbinger Publications.

Chernin, Kim. 1981. *The Obsession: Reflections on the Tyranny of Slenderness*. New York: Harper and Row.

Chrisler, Joan, and Karen Levy. 1990. "The Media Construct a Menstrual Monster: A Content Analysis of PMS Articles in the Popular Press." *Women and Health* 16:89–104.

Chrisman, Bruce. 1989. Testimony before the U.S. Congress, House of Representatives. In *Unqualified Doctors Performing Cosmetic Surgery: Policies and Enforcement: Activities of the Federal Trade Commission—Part I*, 309–332, House, Committee on Small Business, Subcommittee on Regulation, Business Opportunities, and Energy. 101st Cong., 1st sess.

Cocks, Dorothy. 1930. "What about Plastic Surgery?" *Good Housekeeping* 90(6):109ff.

Cole, Celia. 1926. "Lost and Found." *Delineator* 108(6):22ff.

Collins, Mary, and Leslie Zebrowitz. 1995. "The Contributions of Appearance to Occupational Outcomes in Civilian and Military Settings." *Journal of Applied Psychology* 25:129–163.

Conrad, Peter, and Joseph Schneider. 1980. *Deviance and Medicalization: From Badness to Sickness.* St. Louis, Mo.: Mosey.

Costillo, L. Barry. 1985. "Antitrust Enforcement in Health Care: Ten Years after the AMA Suit." *New England Journal of Medicine* 313:901–904.

Courtiss, Eugene. 1986. "Is Surgery by Nonsurgeons in the Public Interest." *Plastic and Reconstructive Surgery* 78:811–812.

Couzens, Gerald. 1992. "Surgically Sculpting Athletic Physiques: Liposuction and Calf and Pectoral Implants." *The Physician and Sportsmedicine.* 20:153–166.

Cox, Carolyn, and Susan Foster. 1990. *The Costs and Benefits of Occupational Regulation.* Washington, D.C.: Federal Trade Commission, Bureau of Economics.

Crane, Mark. 1983. "Competition among Surgeons Takes a Tough New Turn." *Medical Economics* 60:24–29.

Cunningham, Michael, Alan Roberts, Anita Barbee, and Perri Druen. 1995. "'Their Ideas of Beauty Are, on the Whole, the Same as Ours': Consistency and Variability in the Cross–Cultural Perception of Female Physical Attractiveness." *Journal of Personality and Social Psychology* 68:261–279.

Davis, John Staige. 1919. *Plastic Surgery: Its Principles and Practice.* Philadelphia: P. Blaikston's Son & Co.

———. 1926. "Art and Science of Plastic Surgery." *Annals of Surgery* 84:203–210.

Davis, Kathy. 1995. *Reshaping the Female Body: The Dilemma of Cosmetic Surgery.* New York: Routledge.

DeShields, Oscar, Ali Kara, and Erdener Kaynak. 1996. "Source Effects in Purchase Decisions: The Impact of Physical Attractiveness and Accent of Salesperson." *International Journal of Research in Marketing* 13:89–101.

Dickey-Bryant, LeAnne, Gary J. Lautenschlager, Jorge L. Mendoza, and Norman Abrahams. 1986. "Facial Attractiveness and Its Relation to Occupational Success." *Journal of Applied Psychology* 71:16–19.

Dieffenbach, Johann Friedrich. 1845. *Die operative Chirurgie.* Leipzig: Brockhaus.

Dion, Karen. 1972. "Physical Attractiveness and Evaluations of Children's Transgressions." *Journal of Personality and Social Psychology* 24:207–213.

———. 1973. "Young Children's Stereotyping of Facial Attractiveness." *Developmental Psychology* 9:183–188.

Dion, Karen, and Ellen Berscheid. 1974. "Physical Attractiveness and Peer Perception among Children." *Sociometry* 37:1–12.

Dion, Karen, Ellen Berscheid, and Elaine Walster. 1972. "What Is Beautiful Is Good." *Journal of Personality and Social Psychology* 24:285–290.

Dodd, Barbara, and Judi Leahy. 1989. "Facial Prejudice." *American Journal of Mental Retardation* 94: 111.

Dogan, Teoman, Mehmet Bayramicli, and Ayhan Numanoglu. 1997. "Plastic Surgical Techniques in the Fifteenth Century by Serafeddin Sabuncuoglu." *Plastic and Reconstructive Surgery* 99:1775–1779.

Douglas, Mary. 1970. *Natural Symbols: Explorations in Cosmology.* New York: Pantheon Books.

Drogosz, Lisa M., and Paul E. Levy. 1996. "Another Look at the Effects of Appearance, Gender, and Job Type on Performance-Based Decisions." *Psychology of Women Quarterly* 20:437–445.

Dull, Diana, and Candace West. 1991. "Accounting for Cosmetic Surgery: The Accomplishment of Gender." *Social Problems* 38:801–817.

Dutton, Kenneth. 1995. *The Perfectible Body: The Western Ideal of Male Physical Development*. New York: Continuum.

Eagly, Alice, Richard Ashmore, Mona Makhijani, and Laura Longo. 1991. "What Is Beautiful Is Good, But . . ." *Psychological Bulletin* 110:109–128.

Endres, Kathleen. 1995. Introduction to *Women's Periodicals in the United States: Consumer Magazines*, ed. Kathleen Endres and Therese Lueck. Westport, Conn.: Greenwood Press.

Federal Trade Commission. 1975. *Complaint: In Re: American Medical Association, Connecticut State Medical Society, and the New Haven Medical Association*. Docket no. 9064. Washington D.C.: Federal Trade Commission.

———. 1997. *FTC Antitrust Actions in Health Care Services*. Washington D.C.: Federal Trade Commission.

Feingold, Alan. 1990. "Gender Differences in Effects of Physical Attractiveness on Romantic Attraction: A Comparison across Five Research Paradigms." *Journal of Personality and Social Psychology* 59:981–993.

———. 1992. "Good-Looking People Are Not What We Think." *Psychological Bulletin* 111:304–341.

Feingold, Alan, and Ronald Mazzella. 1998. "Gender Differences in Body Image Are Increasing." *Psychological Science* 9:190–195.

Feldstein, Paul. 1996. *The Politics of Health Legislation: An Economic Perspective*. Chicago: Health Administration Press.

Ferguson, Marjorie. 1983. *Forever Feminine: Women's Magazines and the Cult of Femininity*. London: Heinemann Educational Books Ltd.

Finkelstein, Joanne. 1991. *The Fashioned Self*. Cambridge, United Kingdom: Polity Press.

Foubister, Vida. 1999. "Doctors Decry Mandatory Hospitalists." *American Medical News* May 24:16ff.

Fournier, Pierre. 1988. "Who Should Do Syringe Liposculpturing?" *Journal of Dermatologic Surgery and Oncology* 14:1055–1056.

Fox, Bonnie. 1990. "Selling the Mechanized Household: 70 Years of Ads in Ladies Home Journal." *Gender and Society* 4:25–40.

Fredricks, Simon. 1995. "History of the American Society of Plastic and Reconstructive Surgeons." *Plastic and Reconstructive Surgery* 95:1135.

Freedman, Rita. 1986. *Beauty Bound*. Lexington, Mass.: Lexington Books.

Freidson, Eliot. 1980. *Doctoring Together*. Chicago: University of Chicago Press.

———. 1986. *Professional Powers: A Study of the Institutionalization of Formal Knowledge*. Chicago: University of Chicago Press.

———. 1989. *Medical Work in America: Essays on Health Care*. New Haven: Yale University Press.

Freshwater, M. Felix. 1984. "Priorities in Plastic Surgery." *Plastic and Reconstructive Surgery* 73:987–990.

Friedmann, Paul. 1989. "Fragmentation in General Surgery." *Archives of Surgery* 124:1013–1014.

Frieze, Irene, Josephine Olson, and Jane Russell. 1991. "Attractiveness and Income for Men and Women in Management." *Journal of Applied Social Psychology* 21:1039–1057.

Fuerst, Mark. 1983. "Suction-Assisted Lipectomy Attracting Interest." *Journal of the American Medical Association* 249:3004–3005.

Furlan, Silvano, and Riccardo Mazzola. 1995. "Alessandro Benedetti, a Fifteenth Century Anatomist and Surgeon: His Role in the History of Nasal Reconstruction." *Plastic and Reconstructive Surgery* 96:739–743.

Furnham, Adrian, Tina Tan, and Chris McManus. 1997. "Waist-to-Hip Ratio

Preferences for Body Shape: A Replication and Extension." *Personality and Individual Differences* 22:539–549.

Garfield, Bob. 1987. "PR Agency's Idea Rates Bulk Mail." *Advertising Age* 58:40.

Gillespie, Rosemary. 1996. "Women, the Body, and Brand Extension in Medicine: Cosmetic Surgery and the Paradox of Choice." *Women and Health* 24:69–85.

Gilman, Sander. 1999. *Making the Body Beautiful: A Cultural History of Aesthetic Surgery.* Princeton: Princeton University Press.

Glabman, Maureen. 1998. "Spin Doctors." *American Medical News* December 28, 25–27.

Goffman, Erving. 1967. *Interaction Ritual: Essays on Face-to-Face Behavior.* New York: Doubleday.

Goin, John. 1978. "The California Campaign." *Plastic Surgery News* 1(3):3.

Goin, John, and Marcia Goin. 1981. *Changing the Body—Psychological Effects of Plastic Surgery.* Baltimore: Williams & Wilkins.

Goldwyn, Robert. 1977. "Are We Training Surgeons for the Future or the Past?" *Plastic and Reconstructive Surgery* 60:101–103.

———, ed. 1980a. *Long-Term Results in Plastic and Reconstructive Surgery.* Vols. 1 and 2. Boston: Little Brown and Company.

Goldwyn, Robert. 1980b. "The Paraffin Story." *Plastic and Reconstructive Surgery* 65:517–524.

———. 1990a. "History of the American Association of Plastic Surgeons, 1986–1990." *Plastic and Reconstructive Surgery* 87:978–989.

———. 1990b. "When Aesthetic Surgery Is Not Aesthetic." *Plastic and Reconstructive Surgery* 85:949–950.

González-Ulloa, Mario. 1991. "Gluteoplasty: A Ten Year Report." *Aesthetic Plastic Surgery* 15:85–91.

Goode, Erich. 1996. "Gender and Courtship Entitlement: Responses to Personal Ads." *Sex Roles* 334:141–169.

Gorney, Mark. 1980. "The Morning After." *Plastic and Reconstructive Surgery* 66:751–752.

———. 1984. "Mirror, Mirror on the Wall: Presidential Address." *Plastic and Reconstructive Surgery* 74:117–122.

———. 1988. "Patient Selection and Medicolegal Responsibility for the Rhinoplasty Patient." In *Rhinoplasty: Problems and Controversies*, ed. Thomas Rees and Daniel Baker. St. Louis: C. V. Mosby.

———. 1989a. "Who Is Responsible." *Plastic and Reconstructive Surgery* 84:800–801.

———. 1989b. "Advertising in Plastic Surgery: A Position Paper." In *Unqualified Doctors Performing Cosmetic Surgery: Policies and Enforcement Activities of the Federal Trade Commission—Part I*, 206–215, House, Committee on Small Business, Subcommittee on Regulation, Business Opportunities, and Energy. 101st Cong., 1st sess.

Gradinger, Gilbert. 1995. "Update from the American Board of Plastic Surgery." *Plastic Surgery News* 8(3):3.

Green, Cheryl. 1986. "Effects of Counselor and Subject Race and Counselor Physical Attractiveness on Impressions and Expectations of a Female Counselor." *Journal of Counseling Psychology* 33:349–352.

Gross, Stanley. 1984. *Of Foxes and Hen Houses: Licensing and the Health Professions.* Westport, Conn.: Quorum Books.

Gunderson-Warner, Sandi, Lynn Martinez, Israel Martinez, John Carey, Neil Kochenour, and Maury Emery. 1990. "Critical Review of Articles Regarding Pregnancy Exposures in Popular Magazines." *Teratology* 42:469.

Haiken, Beth. 1994. "Plastic Surgery and American Beauty at 1921." *Bulletin History of Medicine* 68:429–453.

Haiken, Elizabeth. 1997. *Venus Envy: A History of Cosmetic Surgery*. Baltimore: The Johns Hopkins University Press.

Hait, Pam. 1994. "History of the American Society of Plastic and Reconstructive Surgeons, Inc., 1931–1994." *Plastic and Reconstructive Surgery* 94:1A–99A.

Halpern, Sydney. 1988. *American Pediatrics: The Social Dynamics of Professionalism, 1880–1980*. Los Angeles: University of California Press.

Hamermesh, Daniel S., and Jeff E. Biddle. 1994. "Beauty and the Labor Market." *American Economic Review* 84:1174–1194.

Hanke, William. 1988. "Liposuction." *Journal of Dermatologic Surgery and Oncology* 14:1051.

Harris, Steven M., and Dean M. Busby. 1998. "Therapist Physical Attractiveness: An Unexplored Influence on Client Disclosure." *Journal of Marital and Family Therapy* 24:251–257.

Haskins, Katherine. 1990. *The Relationship between Weight and Career Payoff for Women*. Ann Arbor: University of Michigan, Dissertation Abstracts International.

Hatala, Mark, and Jill Prehodka. 1996. "Content Analysis of Gay Male and Lesbian Personal Advertisements." *Psychological Reports* 78:371–374.

Hatfield, Elaine, and Susan Sprecher. 1995. "Men's and Women's Preferences in Marital Partners in the United States, Russia, and Japan." *Journal of Cross-Cultural Psychology* 26:728–750.

Henry, Nancy. 1972. "We Zipped It Low This Year: Women's Mags: The Chic Sell." *The Nation* 214 (June 5):710–712.

Hewitt, Kim. 1997. *Mutilating the Body: Identity in Blood and Ink*. Bowling Green, Ohio: Bowling Green State University Popular Press.

Heywood, Leslie. 1998. *Bodymakers: A Cultural Anatomy of Women's Body Building*. New Brunswick, N.J.: Rutgers University Press.

Hildebrandt, Katherine, and Teresa Cannan. 1985. "The Distribution of Caregiver Attention in a Group Program for Young Children." *Child Study Journal* 15:43–55.

Hill, James, and John Peters. 1998. "Environmental Contributions to the Obesity Epidemic." *Science* 280:1371–1374.

Huger, William. 1987. "Presidential Address." *Plastic and Reconstructive Surgery* 80:108–110.

Hughes, Kathleen. 1988. "Body Not Perfect? Nose Too Large? Chest Too Small? Cosmetic Surgeons Compete with Ever-Bolder Ads: Before (Ugh) and After." *Wall Street Journal*. Eastern edition, August 2, 1.

Hugo, Norman. 1982a. "An Update on the Public Education Program of ASPRS." *Plastic Surgery News* 7(2):12.

———. 1982b. "Breaking Down the Communications Barrier." *Plastic Surgery News* 7(9):11.

———. 1997. "Professionalism." Paper presented at the 1997 Canadian Society of Plastic Surgeons Annual Meeting, Calgary, May 21–24.

Iverson, Ronald. 1997. "Plastic Surgery in the United States: Issues and Opportunities." Paper presented at the Canadian Society of Plastic Surgeons Annual Meeting, Calgary, May 21–24.

Jackson, Linda. 1992. *Physical Appearance and Gender: Sociobiological and Sociocultural Perspectives*. Albany: State University of New York Press.

Jackson, Linda, John Hunter, and Carole Hodge. 1995. "Physical Attractiveness and Intellectual Competence: A Meta-Analytic Review." *Social Psychology Quarterly* 58:108–122.

Jarrett, John. 1989. "Quality Assurance in Plastic Surgery." In *Unqualified Doctors Performing Cosmetic Surgery: Policies and Enforcement Activities of the Federal Trade Commission—Part I*, 153–171, House, Committee on Small Business, Subcommittee on Regulation, Business Opportunities, and Energy. 101st Cong., 1st sess.

Johnson, Victor, and Melissa Franklin. 1993. "Is Beauty in the Eye of the Beholder?" *Ethnology and Sociobiology* 14:183–199.

Kaiser, Jocelyn. 1998. "Scientific Panel Clears Breast Implants." *Science* 282: 1963ff.

Kalick, S. Michael, Leslie A. Zebrowitz, Judith H. Langlois, and Robert M. Johnson. 1998. "Does Human Facial Attractiveness Honestly Advertise Health? Longitudinal Data on an Evolutionary Question." *Psychological Science* 9:8–13.

Karraker, Katherine, and Marilyn Stern. 1990. "Infant Physical Attractiveness and Facial Expression: Effects on Adult Perceptions." *Basic and Applied Social Psychology* 11:371–385.

Katz, Shlomo, and Shlomo Kravetz. 1989. "Facial Plastic Surgery for Persons with Down Syndrome: Research Findings and Their Professional and Social Implications." *American Journal on Mental Retardation* 94:101–110.

Kaw, Eugenia. 1993. "Medicalization of Racial Features: Asian American Women and Cosmetic Surgery." *Medical Anthropology Quarterly* 7:74–89.

Kaye, Bernard. 1981. "Quotations, Ruminations, and Illuminations: The State of the Society." *Plastic and Reconstructive Surgery* 68:776–778.

Keller, Kathryn. 1994. *Mothers and Work in Popular American Magazines*. Westport, Conn.: Greenwood Press.

Keller, Matthew, and Robert Young. 1996. "Mate Assortment in Dating and Married Couples." *Personality and Individual Differences* 21:217–221.

Kenealy, Pamela, Neil Frude, and William Shaw. 1988. "Influence of Children's Physical Attractiveness on Teacher Expectations." *The Journal of Social Psychology* 128:373–383.

Kennedy, Janice. 1990. "Determinants of Peer Social Status: Contributions of Physical Appearance, Reputation, and Behavior." *Journal of Youth and Adolescence* 19:233–244.

Kessler, Lauren. 1989. "Women's Magazines' Coverage of Smoking Related Health Hazards." *Journalism Quarterly* 66:316–322ff.

Kirkland, Anna, and Rosemarie Tong. 1996. "Working within Contradiction: The Possibility of Feminist Cosmetic Surgery." *Journal of Clinical Ethics* 7:151–159.

Kisner, Howard. 1993. "A Dilemma." *Plastic and Reconstructive Surgery* 92:1364.

Klein, Alan. 1993. *Little Big Man: Bodybuilding Subculture and Gender Construction*. Albany: State University of New York Press.

Klein, Donald. 1983. "Presidential Address." *Plastic and Reconstructive Surgery* 72:866–867.

Klein, Sarah. 1998. "AMA-Sunbeam Suit Settled." *American Medical News* 41(31):1.

Kmetik, Karen, and David Emmons. 1994. "Physician Advertising: Patterns and Expenditures." In *Socioeconomic Characteristics of Medical Practice*, ed. Martin Gonzalez. Chicago: American Medical Association.

Koot, Hans. 1996. "The Body Image of Children and Adolescents: Implications for Treatment?" In *In the Eye of the Beholder: Ethics and Medical Change of Appearance*, ed. Inez de Beaufort, Medard Hlhorst, and Soren Holm, 134–150. Copenhagen: Scandinavian University Press.

Krizek, Thomas, and Lawrence Ketch. 1994. "The Federal Government and Plastic Surgery Residency." *Annals of Plastic Surgery* 32:84–88.

Lakoff, Robin, and Raquel Scherr. 1984. *Face Value: The Politics of Beauty*. Boston: Routledge.

LaMendola, Bob. 1999. "Cosmetic Surgery Rules Seen as a Retreat." *Sun-Sentinel*. www.Sun-Sentinel/news/plastic.com.

Langlois, Judith. 1986. "From the Eye of the Beholder to Behavioral Reality: Development of Social Behaviors and Social Relations as a Function of Physical Attractiveness." In *Physical Appearance, Stigma, and Social Behaviour: The Ontario Symposium*, Vol. 3, ed. C. Peter Herman, Mark Zanna, and E. Tory Higgins. Hillsdale, N.J.: Erlbaum.

Langlois, Judith, and A. Chris Downs. 1979. "Peer Relations as a Function of Physical Attractiveness." *Child Development* 50:409–418.

Langlois, Judith, Jean Ritter, and Rita Casey. 1995. "Infant Attractiveness Predicts Maternal Behaviors and Attitudes." *Developmental Psychology* 31:464–472.

Langlois, Judith, Jean Ritter, Lori Roggman, and Lesley Vaughn. 1991. "Facial Diversity and Infant Preferences for Attractive Faces." *Developmental Psychology* 27:79–84.

Langlois, Judith, and Lori Roggman. 1990. "Attractive Faces Are Only Average." *Psychological Science* 1:115–121.

Larson, David, Rebecca Anderson, Dawn Maksud, and Brad Grunert. 1994. "What Influences Public Perceptions of Silicone Breast Implants?" *Plastic and Reconstructive Surgery* 94:318–325.

Lerner, Richard, Mary Delaney, Laura Hess, and Jasna Jovanovic. 1990. "Early Adolescent Physical Attractiveness and Academic Competence." *Journal of Early Adolescence* 10:4–20.

Lerner, Richard, Jacqueline Lerner, Laura Hess, and Jacqueline Schwab. 1991. "Physical Attractiveness and Psychosocial Functioning among Early Adolescents." *Journal of Early Adolescence* 11:300–320.

Lewis, John. 1973. *Atlas of Aesthetic Surgery*. Boston: Little Brown and Company.

Lewis, Kathryn, and Margaret Bierly. 1990. "Toward a Profile of the Female Voter: Sex Differences in Perceived Physical Attractiveness and Competence of Political Candidates." *Sex-Roles* 22:1–12.

Loh, Eng Seng. 1993. "The Economic Effects of Physical Appearance." *Social Science Quarterly* 74:420–438.

Longo, Laura C., and Richard D. Ashmore. 1995. "The Looks-Personality Relationship: Global Self-Orientations as Shared Precursors of Subjective Physical Attractiveness and Self-Ascribed Traits." *Journal of Applied Social Psychology* 25:371–398.

Lore, John. 1988. "Presidential Address." *Archives of Otolaryngology—Head and Neck Surgery* 114:385.

Maag, John, Stanley Vasa, Jack Kramer, and Gregory Torrey. 1991. "Teachers' Perceptions of Factors Contributing to Children's Social Status." *Psychological Reports* 69:831–836.

Magazine Industry Marketplace. 1982. *Directory of American Periodical Publishing*. New York: R. R. Bowker Co.

Manstein, Carl. 1987. "Yellow Pages and False Credentials in Plastic Surgery." *Plastic and Reconstructive Surgery* 80:870.

Marder, William, Philip Kletke, Anne Silberger, and Richard Willke. 1988. *Physician Supply and Utilization by Specialty: Trends and Projections.* Chicago, Ill.: American Medical Association.

Margolin, Leslie, and Lynn White. 1987. "The Continuing Role of Physical Attractiveness in Marriage." *Journal of Marriage and the Family* 49:21–27.

Marlowe, Cynthia, Sandra Schneider, and Carnot Nelson. 1996. "Gender and Attractiveness Biases in Hiring Decisions: Are More Experienced Managers Less Biased?" *Journal of Applied Psychology* 81:11–21.

Massachusetts Medical Society. 1961. "Code of Ethics of the Massachusetts Medical Society." In *Massachusetts Medical Society: Its Services and Functions.* Boston: Massachusetts Medical Society.

May, Deborah, and Nancy Turnbull. 1992. "Plastic Surgeons' Opinions of Facial Surgery for Individuals with Down Syndrome." *Mental Retardation* 30: 29–33.

McCracken, Ellen. 1993. *Decoding Women's Magazines from Mademoiselle to Ms.* London: Macmillan.

McCrea, Frances. 1983. "The Politics of Menopause: The 'Discovery' of a Deficiency Disease." *Social Problems* 31:111–123.

McCurdy, John. 1981. *The Complete Guide to Cosmetic Facial Surgery.* Baltimore: Williams & Wilkins.

McNamara, Brooks. 1995. *Step Right Up.* Jackson: University Press of Mississippi.

Mearig, Judith. 1989. "Wanted: Simple Answers to Complex Questions." *American Journal of Mental Retardation* 94:112–113.

Miller, Charles. 1907. *Cosmetic Surgery: The Correction of Featural Imperfections.* Chicago: Oak Printing Company.

Miller, Lois. 1939. "Surgery's Cinderella." *Independent Woman* 18(7):201ff.

Mitteness, Linda. 1983. "Historical Changes in Public Information about the Menopause." *Urban Anthropology* 12:161–179.

Morrow, Paula C., James C. McElroy, Bernard G. Stamper, and Mark A. Wilson. 1990. "The Effects of Physical Attractiveness and Other Demographic Characteristics on Promotion Decisions." *Journal of Management* 16:723–736.

Murray, Joseph, and Thomas Baker. 1970. "Esthetic Surgery and the Plastic Surgeon." *Plastic and Reconstructive Surgery* 46:389.

Murrin, Ruth. 1940. "A New Nose in a Week." *Good Housekeeping* 111(11):82–83.

National Directory of Magazines. 1995. New York: Oxbridge Communications.

Neale, Henry. 1996. "ABMS-ABPS-ABOto Negotiations: Where We've Been and Where We Are Now." *Annals of Plastic Surgery* 36:221–223.

Nell, Kristi, and Nancy Ashton. 1996. "Gender, Self-Esteem, and Perception of Own Attractiveness." *Perceptual and Motor Skills* 83:1105–1106.

Newman, Julius. 1989. Letter to Congressman Wyden. In *Unqualified Doctors Performing Cosmetic Surgery: Policies and Enforcement: Activities of the Federal Trade Commission—Part I*, 300–303, House, Committee on Small Business, Subcommittee on Regulation, Business Opportunities, and Energy. 101st Cong., 1st sess.

Nowak, Linda I., and Judith H. Washburn. 1998. "Patient Sources of Information and Decision Factors in Selecting Cosmetic Surgeons." *Health Care Marketing Quarterly* 15:45–54.

Oliver, Daniel. 1989. Testimony before the U.S. Congress: House of Representatives. In *Unqualified Doctors Performing Cosmetic Surgery: Policies and*

Enforcement: Activities of the Federal Trade Commission—Part II, 29–54, House, Committee on Small Business, Subcommittee on Regulation, Business Opportunities, and Energy. 101st Cong., 1st sess.

Olson, Bradley. 1990. "Physician Specialty Advertising: The Tendency to Deceive?" *Journal of Legal Medicine* 11:351–371.

Owens, Arthur. 1990. "Earnings Make a Huge Breakthrough." *Medical Economics* 67:90–116.

Oxbridge Communication, Inc. 1996. *National Directory of Magazines*. New York: Oxbridge Communication.

Page, Leigh. 1989a. "Should There Be Regulations on Use of MD Specialties?" *American Medical News* September 8:1ff.

———. 1989b. "Specialty Licensure: Sleeper Issue That Could Come Alive." *American Medical News*. September 15: 3ff.

———. 1998. "Will New California Law Hike Surgery Demand?" *American Medical News*. October 19: 1ff.

Page, Randy, Andria Scanlan, and Ola Allen. 1995. "Adolescent Perceptions of Body Weight and Attractiveness: Important Issues in Alcohol and Illicit Drug Use?" *Journal of Child and Adolescent Substance Abuse* 4:43–55.

Palcheff-Wiemer, Mary, Matthew Concannon, Vicki Conn, and Charles Puckett. 1993. "The Impact of the Media on Women with Breast Implants." *Plastic and Reconstructive Surgery* 92:779–785.

Palmer, B. J. 1926. *Selling Yourself*. Davenport, Iowa: Palmer School of Chiropractic.

Palmer, Gretta. 1939. "When Plastic Surgery Is Justified." *Ladies Home Journal* 56(12):20–21.

Patterson, Thomas. 1977. *The Zeis Index and History of Plastic Surgery, 900 b.c.–1863 a.d.* Baltimore: Williams and Wilkins Co.

Patzer, Gordon. 1985. *The Physical Attractiveness Phenomena*. New York: Plenum Press.

Pearl, Robert, Hugh McAllister, and Jay Pruzansky. 1997. "An Economic Analysis of Health Care Reform and Its Implications for Plastic Surgery." *Plastic and Reconstructive Surgery* 99:1–9.

Peirce, Kate. 1990. "A Feminist Theoretical Perspective on the Socialization of Teenage Girls through Seventeen Magazine." *Sex Roles* 23:491–500.

Perrett, D., K. May, and S. Yoshikawa. 1994. "Facial Shape and Judgement of Female Attractiveness." *Nature* 368(6468):239–242.

Peterson, Rex. 1977. "President's Letter." *Plastic Surgery News* 1(2):1.

———. 1978. "Presidential Address: The Spirit of Plastic Surgery." *Plastic and Reconstructive Surgery* 61:490–493.

Petrie, Trent, Laura Austin, Barbara Crowley, Annette Helmcamp, Courtney Johnson, Regan Lester, Rebecca Rogers, Jeff Turner, and Kevin Walbrick. 1996. "Sociocultural Expectations of Attractiveness for Males." *Sex Roles* 35:581–602.

Plastic Surgery News. 1977. "Learning to Field 'Nasty Questions.'" 1(2):7.

———. 1985. "First 'Marketing Your Practice' Seminar Successful." 1(6):1.

———. 1986a. "ASPRS/PSEF Boards Approve New Marketing Department." 2(2):1.

———. 1986b. "Ads Generate Referral Service Calls." 2(5):1.

———. 1986c. "Marketing Conference Meets in Chicago." 2(16):1.

———. 1987a. "ASPRS Awaits AAO–HNS Agreement on Joint Statement." 3(5):1.

———. 1987b. "ASPRS Harnesses Power of the Press." 3(9):1.

————. 1987c. "ASPRS Trying to Shift FTC Focus." 3(9):2.

————. 1987d. "New Practice Building Products Slated for Development." 3(10):1.

————. 1987e. "ASPRS Takes Its Message Directly to the Public." 3(11):1.

————. 1987f. "Release of New Procedures Report Receives Wide-Ranging Media Coverage." 3(16):1.

————. 1988a. "National Audiences Receive Plastic Surgery 'Live.'" 4(1):1.

————. 1988b. "ASPRS Teams Up with *Vogue* in National Health Workshops." 4(8):2.

————. 1988c. "Surgitek to Receive First 'President's Award.'" 4(8):1.

————. 1988d. "Referral Service Receives Increase in Calls about Certification." 4(15):3.

————. 1989a. "Practice Medicine, Not Marketing." 1(1):12.

————. 1989b. "Two Public Education Projects Generate Local, National Interest." 1(1):8.

————. 1989c. "Former President of ASPRS Mark Gorney—FTC." 1(10):3.

————. 1989d. "Regional Advertising Forecast: Selling the Public on Qualified Doctors." 1(11):1ff.

————. 1990a. "AMA Opposed ABMS National Yellow Pages Ad Program." 2(4):1.

————. 1990b. "ASPRS, AAD Find 'Common Ground.'" 2(4):1

————. 1990c. "July 24 *Family Circle* Article on Cosmetic Surgery and Toll Free Number for PSIS." 2(8):9.

————. 1990d. "FTC Speaks out about Board Certification, Medical Advertising." 2(11/12):3.

————. 1991a. "Yellow Pages." 3(3):4.

————. 1991b. "1990 Media Coverage of Plastic Surgery Organizations." 3(4):17.

————. 1991c. "FTC Action Pending: Colorado Passes Law on Medical Advertising." 3(9):1.

————. 1992a. "Members Address Specialty's Needs." 4(4):1ff.

————. 1992b. "Image Audit Offers Mixed Messages." 4(5):1ff.

————. 1992c. "Meeting Its Greatest Challenge: The ASPRS Response to the Silicone Gel Filled Implant Controversy." 4(6): insert.

————. 1993a. "ASPRS and ASAPS Sent Representatives to Meetings of Consumer Groups Opposed to Implants." 5(3):14.

————. 1993b. "Consumer Groups Seek Information, Action for Members." 5(4):14.

————. 1993c. "Accredited Surgical Facilities Offer Protection for Patients." 5(5):1ff.

————. 1993d. "APRS/PSEF 1994 Priorities." 5(5):A8.

————. 1993e. "Avoid Reporters' Snags: Stick to Your Own Agenda." 5(9):5.

————. 1993f. "ASPRS's Annual Meeting Video." 6(10):5.

————. 1994a. "ASPRS Board of Directors Meetings." 7(3):5.

————. 1994b. "Annual Cosmetic Surgery Symposium Continues to Chart 'Cutting Edge.'" 7(4):9.

————. 1994c. "Outcomes Studies Serve as a Tool in Managing Health Reform." 7(6):2–3.

————. 1994d. "ASPRS Encourages Members to Properly Highlight Their Board Certification." 7(9):15.

————. 1994e. "Workforce Study Finds Plastic Surgeon Population Crowded in 2040." 7(10/11):27.

———. 1995a. "Plastic Surgery Information Service Postcards Increase Routes, Frequency of Patient Referrals." 8(1):19.

———. 1995b. "The Conjoint Symposium on Contemporary Head and Neck Reconstruction." 8(4)25.

———. 1995c. "ASPRS/PSEF Report to Membership." 8(5):A2.

———. 1995d. "ASPRS Workforce Study." 8(6):4.

———. 1995e. "1994 Procedural Statistics Update." 8(7):16.

———. 1995f. "Plastic Surgery Practice Update." 8(8):3.

———. 1996a. "July 1 Deadline for Accreditation of California's Ambulatory Surgery Facilities." 9(1):8.

———. 1996b. "Report on the National Endowment." 9(3):23.

———. 1996c. "Strategic Planning Identifies Goals and Impacts." 9(3):26.

———. 1997a. "Campaign Launches: Plastic Surgery Educational Campaign Ads Hit Magazines, TV." 9b(1):1.

———. 1997b. "National Endowment Funds Reduction Outcomes Study." 9b(5):2.

———. 1997c. "ASPRS Monitors Discussions on Joint Plastic Surgery Certification." 9b(6):16.

———. 1997d. "Integrate Practice Marketing with Society's PSEC Programs." 9b(6):29.

———. 1997e. "2nd Conjoint Rhinoplasty Symposium." 9b(6):17.

———. 1997f. "1997 Annual Scientific Meeting." 9b(7):1.

———. 1997g. "New AMS Patient Financing Program Launched." 9b(7):16.

———. 1997h. "Plastic Surgery Update Supplement." 9b(7):33.

Polhemus, Ted, and Housk Randall. 1996. *The Customized Body*. New York: Serpent's Tail.

Pope, Harrison, Roberto Olivardia, Amanda Gruber, and John Borowiecki. 1999. "Evolving Ideals of Male Body Image as Seen through Action Toys." *International Journal of Eating Disorders* 26:65–72.

Prager, Linda. 1999. "Upping the Certification Ante." *American Medical News*, June 7, 1ff.

Pueschel, Siegfried. 1988. "Facial Plastic Surgery for Children with Down Syndrome." *Developmental Medicine and Child Neurology* 30:536–549.

Randolph, Lillian. 1997. *Physician Characteristics and Distribution in the U.S.* Chicago, Ill.: American Medical Association.

Reade, Julia, and Richard Ratzan. 1987. "Yellow Professionalism: Advertising by Physicians in the Yellow Pages." *New England Journal of Medicine* 316:1315–1319.

Reader's Guide to Periodical Literature. 1900–1999. New York: H. W. Wilson Co.

Reddick, Lovett. 1991. "From a Broken Soapbox: Misadventures in Plastic Surgery." *Plastic and Reconstructive Surgery* 87:941–945.

Rees, Thomas. 1986. "Discussion of W. Earle Matory Jr. and Edward Falces, 'Non-Caucasian Rhinoplasty.'" *Plastic and Reconstructive Surgery* 77:252.

———. 1991. "The Surgery of Aesthetics: A Modern Dilemma." *Aesthetic Plastic Surgery* 15:99–104.

Rees, Thomas, and D. Wood-Smith. 1973. *Cosmetic Facial Surgery*. Philadelphia: W. B. Saunders Company.

Regan, Thomas. 1985. "Aesthetic Facial Surgery in the Otolaryngology Program." *Archives of Otolaryngology* 111:141.

Reingen, Peter, and Jerome Kernan. 1993. "Social Perception and Interpersonal Influence: Some Consequences of the Physical Attractiveness Stereotype in a Personal Selling Setting." *Journal of Consumer Psychology* 2:25–38.

Reissman, Catherine. 1983. "Women and Medicalization." *Social Policy* 14:3–18.

Ring, Malvin. 1991. "The History of Maxillofacial Prosthetics." *Plastic and Reconstructive Surgery* 87:174–184.

Ritter, Jean, Rita Casey, and Judith Langlois. 1991. "Adults' Responses to Infants Varying in Appearance of Age and Attractiveness." *Child Development* 62:68–82.

Ritts, Vicki, Miles Patterson, and Mark Tubbs. 1992. "Expectations, Impressions, and Judgments of Physically Attractive Students: A Review." *Review of Educational Research* 62:413–426.

Rogers, Blair. 1976. "The Development of Aesthetic Plastic Surgery: A History." *Aesthetic Plastic Surgery* 1:2–22.

———. 1988. "History of Oculoplastic Surgery: The Contributions of Plastic Surgery." *Aesthetic Plastic Surgery* 12:129–152.

Romano, Shelia, and James Bordiere. 1989. "Physical Attractiveness Stereotypes and Students' Perceptions of College Professors." *Psychological Reports* 64:1099–1102.

Ruberg, Robert. 1994. "A Proposal for Achieving Reduction in the Number of Plastic Surgery Residents Completing Training Each Year." *Annals of Plastic Surgery* 32:80–81.

Rubin, Leonard. 1982. "Advertising and PR Agents." *Plastic and Reconstructive Surgery* 69:117–118.

Ruggiero, Josephine, and Louise Weston. 1985. "Work Options for Women in Women's Magazines: The Medium and the Message." *Sex Roles* 12: 535–547.

Rynes, Sara, and Barry Gerhart. 1990. "Interviewer Assessments of Applicant 'Fit': An Exploratory Investigation." *Personnel Psychology* 43:13–35.

Sanders, Clinton. 1989. *Customizing the Body: The Art and Culture of Tattooing.* Philadelphia: Temple University Press.

Santoni-Rugiu, Paolo, and Riccardo Mazzola. 1997. "Leonardo Fioravanti (1517–1588): A Barber-Surgeon Who Influenced the Development of Reconstructive Surgery." *Plastic and Reconstructive Surgery* 99: 570–575.

Sarwer, David B., Thomas A. Wadden, Michael J. Pertschuk, and Linton A. Whitaker. 1998. "The Psychology of Cosmetic Surgery: A Review and Reconceptualization." *Clinical Psychology Review* 18:1–22.

Saul, Ann. 1996. "Plastic Surgeons Examine Group Practice Options." *Plastic Surgery News* 9(1):1.

Schalk, Deborah. 1988. "The History of Augmentation Mammoplasty." *Plastic Surgical Nursing* 8:88–90.

Schulte, Fred, and Jenni Bergal. 1998. *Cosmetic Surgery: The Hidden Dangers.* www.sun-sentinel.com/news/plastic.

Selz, Michael. 1997. "Lenders Find Niche in Cosmetic Surgery That Isn't Insured." *Wall Street Journal*, Eastern Edition, January 15, PA1ff.

Sherman, James. 1989. "'Facial Plastic Surgery for Persons with Down Syndrome': What Are the Results and Whose Interests Prevail?" *American Journal of Mental Retardation* 94:114–115.

Sigall, Harold, and David Landy. 1973. "Radiating Beauty: Effects of Having a Physically Attractive Partner on Person Perception." *Journal of Personality and Social Psychology* 28:218–224.

Simmons Market Research Bureau, Inc. 1994. *The Simmons Study of Media and Markets, Publications: Total Audiences.* New York: Simmons Market Research Bureau.

Simons, Robert, and T. Susan Hill. 1989. *Coming of Age: A Twenty-Fifth An-*

niversary of the American Academy of Facial Plastic and Reconstructive Surgery. Washington, D.C.: American Academy of Facial Plastic and Reconstructive Surgery.

Singer, Eleanor, and Phyllis Endreny. 1987. "Reporting Hazards: Their Benefits and Costs." *Journal of Communications* 37:10.

Singh, Devendra. 1993. "Adaptive Significance of Female Physical Attractiveness: Role of Waist-to-Hip Ratio." *Journal of Personality and Social Psychology* 65:293–307.

———. 1994. "Is Thin Really Beautiful and Good? Relationship between Waist-to-Hip Ratio (WHR) and Female Attractiveness." *Personality and Individual Differences* 16:123–132.

———. 1995. "Female Judgment of Male Attractiveness and Desirability for Relationships: Role of Waist-to-Hip Ratio and Financial Status." *Journal of Personality and Social Psychology* 69:1089–1101.

Singh, Devendra, and Robert Young. 1995. "Body Weight, Waist-to-Hip Ratio, Breasts, and Hips: Role in Judgments of Female Attractiveness and Desirability for Relationships." *Ethology and Sociobiology* 16:483–507.

Smith, Jane, V. Ann Waldorf, and David Trembath. 1990. "'Single White Male Looking for Thin, Very Attractive . . .'" *Sex Roles* 23:675–685.

Sprecher. 1989. "The Importance to Males and Females of Physical Attractiveness, Earning Potential, and Expressiveness in Initial Attraction." *Sex Roles* 21:591–607.

Starr, Paul. 1982. *The Social Transformation of American Medicine.* New York: Basic Books.

Steinem, Gloria. 1990. "Sex, Lies, and Advertising." *Ms.* 1(7/8):18–28.

Stephan, Cookie, and Judith Langlois. 1984. "Baby Beautiful: Adult Attributions of Infant Competence as a Function of Infant Attractiveness." *Child Development* 55:576–585.

Stevens, Rosemary. 1999. "Professional Competence and Board Certification." Paper presented at the Conference of the American Board of Medical Specialties, Chicago, March.

Stott, Martha. 1997a. "ASPRS Advertising Campaign Reaches Consumers." *Plastic Surgery News* 9b(5):6.

———. 1997b. "Advertising Builds Public Recognition: PSEC Extended through '97—and Beyond." *Plastic Surgery News* 9b(6):1.

Straatsma, Clarence. 1932. "Plastic Surgery: Its Uses and Limitations." *New York State Journal of Medicine* 32:254.

Strathern, Andrew. 1996. *Body Thoughts.* Ann Arbor: University of Michigan Press.

Strauss, Ronald, Reuven Feuerstein, Yael Mintzker, Yaakov Rand, and Menachem-Ron Wexler. 1989. "Ordinary Faces? Down Syndrome, Facial Surgery, Active Modification, and Social Perceptions." *American Journal of Mental Retardation* 94:115–118.

Stricker, Michel, Jacques Meulen, B. Vander Raphad, and Riccardo Mazzola. 1990. *Craniofacial Malformations.* Edinburgh: Churchill Livingstone.

Struckman-Johnson, Cindy, and David Struckman-Johnson. 1994. "Men's Reactions to Hypothetical Female Sexual Advances: A Beauty Bias in Responses to Sexual Coercion." *Sex Roles* 31:387–405.

Sullivan, Deborah, and Rose Weitz. 1988. *Labor Pains: Modern Midwives and Homebirth.* New Haven: Yale University Press.

Taylor, John. 1995. "The Long, Hard Days of Dr. Dick." *Esquire* 124(9):120–130.

Thornhill, Randy, and Steven Gangestad. 1993. "Human Facial Beauty: Averageness, Symmetry, and Parasite Resistance." *Human Nature* 4:237–269.

Trotta, Geri. 1960. "The Wish to Be Beautiful." *Harper's Bazaar* 101(6):126.

Tuchman, Gaye, Arlene Kaplan Daniels, and James Benet. 1978. *Hearth and Home: Images of Women in the Mass Media.* New York: Oxford University Press.

Udry, Richard, and Bruce Eckland. 1984. "Benefits of Being Attractive: Differential Payoffs for Men and Women." *Psychological Reports* 54:47–56.

Umberson, Debra, and Michael Hughes. 1987. "The Impact of Physical Attractiveness in Achievement and Psychological Well-Being." *Social Psychology Quarterly* 50:227–236.

Updegraff, H. K. 1938. "The Fall and Rise of Plastic Surgery." Paper presented at the Society of *Plastic and Reconstructive Surgery* in Philadelphia, November 5.

U.S. Bureau of the Census. 1984. *Statistical Abstract of the United States: 1984.* Washington D.C.

———. 1990. *Statistical Abstract of the United States: 1990.* Washington D.C.

———. 1998. *Statistical Abstract of the United States: 1998.* Washington D.C.

———. 1999. *1998 Statistical Abstract of the United States.* Washington D.C. www.census.gov.

U.S. Department of Health and Human Services. 1980. *Summary Report of the Graduate Medical Educational National Advisory Committee.* Washington, D.C.

———. 1983. *Health: United States,* 1982. Washington D.C.

U.S. House. 1989a. Committee on Small Business, Subcommittee on Regulation, Business Opportunities, and Energy. *Unqualified Doctors Performing Cosmetic Surgery: Policies and Enforcement: Activities of the Federal Trade Commission—Part I.* 101st Cong., 1st sess.

———. 1989b. Committee on Small Business, Subcommittee on Regulation, Business Opportunities, and Energy. *Unqualified Doctors Performing Cosmetic Surgery: Policies and Enforcement: Activities of the Federal Trade Commission—Part II.* 101st Cong., 1st sess.

———. 1989c. Committee on Small Business, Subcommittee on Regulation, Business Opportunities, and Energy. *Unqualified Doctors Performing Cosmetic Surgery: Policies and Enforcement: Activities of the Federal Trade Commission—Part III.* 101st Cong., 1st sess.

———. 1990. Committee on Government Operations, Subcommittee on Human Resources and Intergovernmental Relations. *Is the FDA Protecting Patients from the Dangers of Silicone Breast Implants?* 102nd Cong., 2nd sess.

Vanderford, Marsha, David Smith, and Tonja Olive. 1995. "The Image of Plastic Surgeons in News Media Coverage of the Silicone Breast Implant Controversy." *Plastic and Reconstructive Surgery* 96:521–538.

Veblen, Thorstein. 1899. *Theory of the Leisure Class: An Economic Study of Institutions.* New York: Macmillan Company.

Vener, Arthur, and Lawrence Krupka. 1986. "Over-the-Counter Drug Advertising in Gender-Oriented Popular Magazines." *Journal of Drug Education* 16:367–381.

Walsh, Richard. 1927. "The Divine Right to Look Human." *Woman's Home Companion* 54(10):29–30.

Walt, Alexander. 1986. "Implications of Fragmentation in Surgery on Graduate Training and Certification." *American College of Surgeons Bulletin* 71:2–5ff.

Webster, George. 1977. "Whatever Happened to Ethics?" *Plastic and Reconstructive Surgery* 60:100.

Webster, Richard. 1984. "Cosmetic Surgery: Its Past, Present, and Future." *Journal of Cosmetic Surgery* 1:3–14.

Welter, Barbara. 1973. "The Cult of True Womanhood: 1820–1860." In *The Underside of American History: Other Readings*, ed. Thomas R. Frazier. New York: Harcourt Brace Jovanovich.

Wertz, Richard, and Dorothy Wertz. 1977. *Lying In: A History of Childbirth in America*. New York: Schocken Books.

Weston, Louise, and Josephine Ruggiero. 1985. "The Popular Approach to Women's Health Issues: A Content Analysis of Women's Magazines in the 1970s." *Women and Health* 10: 47–62.

Wheeler, Ladd, and Youngmee Kim. 1997. "What Is Beautiful Is Culturally Good: The Physical Attractiveness Stereotype Has Different Content in Collectivistic Cultures." *Personality and Social Psychology Bulletin* 23:795–800.

Williams, Richard, M. Elizabeth Gee, and Edward Grimmer. 1978. *Memorandum: Recommendation That Complaint Issue against the American Society of Plastic and Reconstructive Surgeons, Inc., for Violation of Section 5 of the Federal Trade Commission Act by Excluding Competitors*. Washington, D.C.: Bureau of Competition, Federal Trade Commission.

Wolf, Naomi. 1991. *The Beauty Myth: How Images of Beauty Are Used against Women*. New York: William Morrow and Company.

Yellow Pages Publishers Association. 1988. *1987–1988 YPPA Study on the Role of the Yellow Pages in the Purchase Decision on 24 Product/Service Categories*. Westfield, N.J.: Statistical Research Inc.

Zebrowitz, Leslie. 1997. *Reading Faces: Windows to the Soul?* Boulder, Colo.: Westview Press.

Zebrowitz, Leslie, Mary Ann Collins, and Ranjana Dutta. 1998. "The Relationship between Appearance and Personality across the Life Span." *Personality and Social Psychology Bulletin* 24:736–749.

Zebrowitz, Leslie, Joann Montepare, and Hoon Koo Lee. 1993. "They Don't All Look Alike: Individual Impressions of Other Racial Groups." *Journal of Personality and Social Psychology* 65:85–101.

Zebrowitz, Leslie, Karen Olson, and Karen Hoffman. 1993. "The Stability of Babyfaceness and Attractiveness across the Lifespan." *Journal of Personality and Social Psychology* 64:453–466.

Zebrowitz, Leslie, Luminita Voinescu, and Mary Ann Collins. 1996. "'Wide-Eyed' and 'Crooked Faced': Determinants of Perceived and Real Honesty across the Life Span." *Personality and Social Psychology Bulletin* 22:1250–1269.

Zook, Elvin. 1993. "Where Should the Battle to Improve Specialty's Image Be Fought and Won?" *Plastic Surgery News* 6(11):2.

Zuckerman, Miron, Kunitate Miyake, and Charlotte Elkin. 1995. "Effects of Attractiveness and Maturity of Face and Voice on Interpersonal Impressions." *Journal of Research in Personality* 29:253–272.

Index

About the Author

Deborah A. Sullivan teaches sociology at Arizona State University. She is the coauthor of *Labor Pains: Modern Midwives and Home Birth.*